FREDERICK CHRISTOPHER, M.D.

Emeritus Professor of Surgery, Northwestern University Medical School

One Surgeon's Practice

W. B. SAUNDERS COMPANY

Philadelphia   *1957*   *London*

TO

D. W. C.

Preface

IN this book are recorded some personal observations and experiences not only in the preparation for and the development of an average general surgical practice, but also in the daily practical and detailed conduct of such professional work. Included are anecdotes and illustrative examples.

It is hoped that the information here presented may be of interest to those who wish to obtain a picture of what a general surgical practice may be, especially those who are contemplating the study of medicine. It is intended, moreover, to be of help to medical students, interns, residents, practicing surgeons and general practitioners.

Included are discussions of the selection of a medical school, choice of a locality in which to practice, hospital staff and society memberships, the conduct of the surgeon in the operating room, the teaching of medical students and house officers, medical research, conversations with patients and relatives regarding operations and regarding cancer, medical writing, surgical fees and surgical pitfalls.

FREDERICK CHRISTOPHER

Winnetka, Illinois
July, 1957

Contents

CHAPTER I

Preparation for a Surgical Practice

THE decision to study medicine is made with difficulty in some cases and easily in others. Frequently the ambition to become a doctor is aroused at an early age but, as in my own case, sometimes not until after graduation from college. This ambition evolves from a combination of many factors, such as the character, objectives and industriousness of one's parents, one's environment, one's intelligence and one's concept of the practice of medicine.

Usually a young man takes up medicine because of admiration of a certain physician, either a relative or a friend, or has appreciated the kindness shown to him during an illness by a physician and is impelled to try to imitate that physician. Regardless of the information he may have, a young man may feel intensely interested in the subject of medicine or may be attracted by its occasionally dramatic aspects portrayed in movies and on television and by the highly colored accounts found in some novels. In the early days, a physician was looked up to in his community as one of the few outstanding men of the region. Admittedly, this social prestige has been diminishing. No young man should contemplate a career of medicine if he thinks he will have an easy life. Nor should he enter medicine in anticipation of great financial rewards, for he almost certainly will not obtain them. Fortunate is the young man who has his mind definitely made up before going to college or shortly thereafter. While such a decision is usually made on an emotional and idealistic rather than factual basis, it is usually unshakable.

To the young man trying to make a decision as to his life's work, certain books, which likely will be more fully appreciated and better evaluated during college years than in high school, may be helpful. The first of these guides is *A History of Medicine* by Ralph H. Major.[1] Another is *A Surgeon's Life* by J. M. T. Finney.[2] Older but still valuable is *Aequanimitas and Other Essays* by William Osler.[3] In 1954 Noah D. Fabricant[4] published *Why We Became Doctors,* in which he gives, in their own words, the reasons why fifty doctors selected medicine as a career.

Any one who contemplates medicine as a career will learn much from reading an admirable anthology entitled *400 Years of a Doctor's Life.*[5] The authors say:

"In this book the doctor's life is revealed in all its aspects, so that reading it, you—the patient—may now examine the doctor. For such a scrutiny there is no better source of information than the doctor himself. Out of many ventures in medical autobiography made during the past four centuries there have been chosen those passages which are most revealing of the medical human being in the round— that convey something of the substance and marrow of what it means to be a doctor. The aim is to present an informal portrait which will show the doctor not only as the Great Healer or Great Scientist (though these aspects are not neglected) but also as a citizen of everyman's world. To achieve this aim, more than eighty personalities have been selected from among men and women who have made significant contributions to the literature of medical autobiography. . . . Here you meet doctors from Austria, Canada, France, Germany, Great Britain, Italy, Russia, Spain, Sweden, Switzerland, and the United States."

Certainly, to witness an operation has slight value. It is a mere spectacle, since the novice cannot possibly understand what it is all about. The first operation that I witnessed made me somewhat ill. Similarly, a visit to a dissecting room is unpleasant and does not give any inkling regarding the practice of medicine.

I would recommend that a young man be shown the workings of an outpatient department in a medical school or a large hospital. There he will see unfortunate, sometimes dirty, ignorant people whom he must later help while they, in turn, help him to learn about medicine. If he feels kindly toward them and if he is interested in the fact that these people have problems which he, as a doctor, should be able to help solve, he is on the right road. He should talk to some medical students in order to obtain an idea of the intensity of their studies and the time-consuming work required, keeping in mind, meanwhile, that any student a few years older than himself will probably be tempted to affect an air of cynical intellectual omnipotence. A friendly visit with a successful young practitioner will aid greatly, particularly if the latter leads him to realize the deep concern for his patients which often lies beneath a doctor's cheery, confident manner. Best of all is a talk with an older physician, one who has had a fine career and who has the patience to discuss matters with him. Such a man may help him evaluate his interests, motives and capacities. Such a conversation might clarify the fact that a studious mind is essential, and while aggressive confidence, cheerfulness and a pleasing personality are splendid allies, they are never substitutes for intelligence.

A university degree is a prerequisite for the study of medicine. I have a firm belief that during the university period the student must learn to think and to make decisions and should become enriched as much as possible by the cultural subject matter of the humanities. Once in medical school, he must apply himself to such intensive and highly specialized courses that there is no opportunity for such studies. Only the minimum amount of time should be spent on so-called "premedical" work in order to comply with medical school entrance requirements. Of course, elementary chemistry is a necessity, and physics, botany and zoology are legitimate preparatory courses. Frankly, however, I hope that the stress on science requirements will be decreased. Usually much of the liberal arts work in the sciences is repeated more intensively and more practically in medical school. I am confident that the ultimate product—a surgeon—will be greatly profited by studying history, English literature, economics, mathematics, philosophy, astronomy and geology before entering medical school.

The currently proposed plan to make college and medical school an eight-year unit in which the so-called "memory" courses, such as anatomy and physiology, are taught in the first years and the so-called "reasoning" courses are taught in the last years, impresses me as a rather precarious experiment. The first pitfall lies in the assumption that only those students who decide at high school graduation on a medical career should be accepted. The second pitfall is the wide separation in time of the study of anatomy and physiology from the study of clinical surgery and medicine.

Will Mayo[6] once said:

> "If one of the years which is given to pre-medical work in our universities could be given to social education, it would help the physician understand the psychology of the emotional field. Ability to evaluate emotional reactions and their relation to society would often be of greater value to him and to the patient than the so-called higher pre-medical culture."

In a comprehensive report on premedical education in the United States,[7] three eminent deans, Aura E. Severinghaus, associate dean of Columbia University's faculty of medicine, William E. Cadbury, Jr., of Haverford, and Dean Emeritus Harry Carman, of Columbia College, deprecated the emphasis upon science courses and stated their belief that colleges and medical schools are graduating too many doctors with "little or no interest in the cultural implications of their profession, much less in those things which would enable them to formulate for themselves a satisfying philosophy of life."

The university that is attended—if it is possible to have a choice—should be the one with the most stimulating and interesting instructors. Who could fail to profit from the inspiration of such men as the late William Lyon Phelps, of Yale, and Gilbert Highet, of Columbia. Moreover, the student should choose, if possible, a university where the level of undergraduate intelligence is at least equal to his own, and preferably higher. Such a university should give outlet to the exuberance of youth by means of sports in which all participate and should minimize the spectacles in which the majority of the students merely observe the games (in spite of the fact that the spectacular contests are financially important to many universities). Where the fraternity system is strongly developed, the student will probably benefit by becoming a member of one of the leading groups, since a good fraternity often adds to one's education in the humanities. Unless abundantly subsidized, the student usually is wise not to marry while in college and medical school, although it is easy to cite notable exceptions to such counsel.

Never again in his life will the student have such an opportunity to acquaint himself with great thoughts and great facts and to acquire valuable habits of mental discipline and drill. To the extent that he avails himself of these opportunities, will his character and

4

his usefulness be strengthened and enriched. It seems best to admonish the student not to permit valuable opportunities to be missed because of excessive participation in such feverish student activities as "rushing," parades, rallies, class politics and the like. Of course, a certain amount of fun and of physical activity is necessary, but these should have their proper place. It is often desirable in the summer months to build up physical strength and health by means of outdoor activities. Those who can take a walking or bicycle trip in Europe are fortunate.

The choice of a medical school may be influenced by cost and location. The tuition, while steadily increasing, does not approximate the cost of educating a doctor. The 1953 Annual Report of the American Medical Education Foundation gives the total four-year cost of training a typical medical student as $13,356.00. This figure was based on 1948 teaching costs. The most important factor, however, is the quality of instruction, which in turn is dependent upon many factors. A school must have enough funds so that it can secure distinguished teachers and provide them with the most up-to-date and adequate buildings and equipment. A medical school should be located in a city of sufficient size that it has abundant patient-teaching material in outpatient departments and in the hospital. The growth of health insurance plans, both private and governmental, is raising some problems for medical instruction which will have to be solved. The institution should have a satisfactory record for its graduates in state board examinations and in their further progress.

In the clinical branches, there should not be too many full-time professors, as they tend to become more academic and less practical if they do not actually engage in some private practice. If possible, young instructors should be paid a small salary and should teach on the basis of their own experience, supplemented by textbooks. It is lamentable that the age of medical heroes seems to be passing. The reverence with which students at Johns Hopkins fifty years ago looked up to and admired Osler, Barker and Finney seldom finds its counterpart now. Whenever Barker held a clinic, the largest amphitheater was always crowded to capacity. His urbane manner, his clear exposition and his dignified bearing left an unforgettable impression on his audience.

The method of selecting the heads of departments in medical schools has a definite bearing on the quality of instruction. Often these men are chosen on the basis of highly praiseworthy research work or prestige from the development of a technical skill but may be deficient in the administrative and pedagogic ability necessary to coordinate and vivify teaching so as to "manufacture" the best physicians. A prospective medical student will do well to study the 56th "Annual Report on Medical Education in the United States and Canada" prepared by the Council on Medical Education and Hospitals of the American Medical Association.[8]

Seventy-five years ago students seldom examined or talked to any patients. That obvious discrepancy in teaching has been largely overcome since the pioneer efforts of Osler and other great leaders. In the fourth year and usually also in the third year, a medical student when acting as a "clinical clerk" studies a patient much as does a physician, only in much more detail. Physical diagnosis is taught on patients in the third year and even, to a degree, in the second year. However, the pendulum is swinging too far, on the false theory that if some clinical work is good, a great amount is better. It must not become a medical school fashion or supposed mark of progressive methods to increase and to accelerate this student-patient contact and the performance of minor mechanical procedures at the expense of solid study of the fundamentals detailed in the textbooks. At present the clinical approach is increasing almost torrentially in the fourth year, intern year and residency period.

Gibbon[9] wisely observes: "As education is a life-long process, it seems obvious that if a medical student fails to acquire the ability to educate himself, he will be a poor physician throughout his professional life."

Michael Davis[10] says:

"Preparation for medicine has been oriented to the growing subject matter of a vocation rather than the changing needs of a society. One is led to suspect that the reason for this situation goes back to the control of medical education by specialists who have been thinking about teaching their subject matter, instead of by educators who view the student and the educational process as a whole, and whose objective is to prepare men and women for professional service to society and for well-adjusted personal lives."

The subject matter of medicine has become so complex and voluminous that no student can master all of it, even with the most indefatigable concentration. Therefore, it is usually unwise to

6

permit the undergraduate medical student to engage in extracurricular research. Often his time and energy are solicited by an instructor to help complete a task that may enhance the instructor's reputation. The student hopes to gain favor, but it is at the expense of time taken from study of the vast, solid subject matter of medicine. In many institutions every student seems to be regarded as a potential research worker, or at least a test-tube cleaner and animal *diener* for an instructor's project. It is argued that the weaker students will fall by the wayside. To my way of thinking, the truly dedicated research workers are few and far between. In order to select these men, it might not be too whimsical to have an American Board of Research, which will determine just who shall be permitted and encouraged to engage in research.

The proponents of research by medical students maintain that such endeavors cultivate an inquiring mind and logical reasoning. Admittedly, it often does this to a certain extent and trains the student in attacking and completing an *Arbeit*. Nevertheless, a physician's prime function is the care of sick people, which entails maximum acquaintance with a vast and rapidly increasing medical storehouse of knowledge and the study of people themselves so that the acquired knowledge can be correctly applied. The student will soon be clothed in authority, and he must do his utmost during his medical course to prepare himself to fulfil the responsibility and obligation so that he will not be found wanting.

When the student enters medical school, he finds his work, associations and environment so different from what he has experienced in the past that he may begin to think he has made a mistake. This was certainly true in my own case. I knew no one at Johns Hopkins except Dean Howell when I went to the first meeting of the new students in a dreary old amphitheater in an unprepossessing building in the older part of Baltimore. Dr. Finney addressed the assembly in ringing, forceful tones: "If any man in this room has the slightest hesitation about his decision to study medicine, let him leave at once!" I almost did.

Undoubtedly the thoughtful choice and cultivation of friendships and associations with serious-minded fellow students will prove helpful in study and discussion. I have always been aware of my good fortune in having as a roommate Admont H. Clark, who had a fine character and great intellectual strength. His parents were missionaries in Japan, and he had worked his way through Oberlin College, somehow finding time to play football and becoming a skilled violinist. A genuine interest in research possessed him, and in 1918 he was perfusing the pancreas in experimental animals. Had not influenza ended his life that year, it is not at all unlikely that he might have been the one to discover insulin.

All medical students are apt to overexpend their physical reserves. It is well for them to assign a definite time for physical exercise and recreation and to be sure of the proper amount of sleep.

It is now customary to grant the degree of Doctor of Medicine upon the completion of the fourth year of medical training. Early in the fourth year the student tries to inform himself as to the character and availability of various types of internships in his own city and elsewhere about the country. He then applies for an internship in three or four, indicating his order of choice. After an elaborate joint selection machinery has functioned, he is assigned a certain internship. The average student is prone to place the highest value upon an internship where he has the maximum authority in the treatment of patients and where he is permitted to do the most procedures of various kinds. As a consequence, the large charity hospitals have always been popular. I am inclined to question the wisdom of this line of reasoning.

While the matter is something that each man will have to decide for himself, to my mind the essential qualifications for a good internship include the following: First, and by far most important, are the character and intellectual ability of the men on the attending staff. These men should be most keenly aware of advances in medical knowledge and should be actually participating in research work. Usually the attending staff teach in a medical school, but a man may be an excellent teacher without being a member of a medical school faculty. The attending men should have the highest ethical standards as well as skill in the management of patients in their various specialties. It is difficult for the medical student to appreciate that he will learn far more by observing an expert physician in his daily practice of medicine than he will by attempting the actual care of patients himself if he is poorly supervised and especially if he is unsupervised.

The so-called "rotating" internship seems the best, since the intern will spend a certain amount of time on each of the various specialties and subspecialties, including general internal medicine, infectious diseases, pediatrics, dermatology, neurology and psychiatry, general surgery, orthopedic surgery, otolaryngology, ophthalmology, neurological surgery, urology, proctology, obstetrics, gynecology, anesthesiology, pathology, roentgenology, radiation therapy and oral surgery. It is extremely important that the intern have a term of service in the accident or emergency room and also in the outpatient department.

The intern's work is more demanding physically and mentally than anything he has previously experienced. He now has serious responsibilities in the actual care of patients. Toward them he should be unfailingly considerate, patient and kindly despite frequent provocation to be otherwise. He must never allow himself to regard patients simply as individuals put there for his special benefit and from whom he must learn as much as possible. If he does his utmost to serve his patients well, then he will indeed learn, in so doing, to be a good doctor. His work must be accurate, complete and intelligent, but, of course, there is never time enough in which to do everything. The intern must carefully write a complete history of each new patient, make a thorough examination, record his findings and make a tentative diagnosis.

Each day the intern endeavors to meet his attending man promptly when the latter arrives at the hospital, make rounds with him and write such orders as the attending man requests. During the entire twenty-four hours of each day he must immediately respond to all manner of calls, although some of them may prove to be quite unnecessary, regarding any changes in a patient's condition, and he will always try to keep the attending man informed of such changes. If he is unable to reach the attending man, he must confer with a resident or a superior on the house staff or act on his own responsibility. He should always be in the operating room promptly for the beginning of an operation and be constantly on the alert to try to minimize the patient's apprehension and discomfort. He later writes "progress notes," that is, brief notes in the chart telling of the course of the patient's illness. He should be uniformly courteous to all nurses, supervisors, nurse aids, ward helpers and other hospital personnel. Throughout his internship he should bear in mind that a record is being kept of his activities and will be the basis for replies to future requests for references for him when he is applying for other work. Needless to say, the best residencies are awarded to the interns who have made the best records.

During, or even before, the internship year, the young doctor will have to decide whether he is going to begin general practice immediately on completion of his internship, take a salaried position of some kind or prepare himself for a specialty. General practice, or "general medicine," as it is now frequently called, offers many attractions. In an excellent article, Clark[11] of Andover, Massachusetts, discusses the work of the "generalist" in urban, suburban, small-city, semirural and rural practices and defines the scope of each.

Fifty years ago it was usually thought unwise for a doctor to specialize until after he had completed five to ten years of general practice. Much can be said for the basic wisdom of such a plan, but only a few men are able to achieve the financial means or have the energy to break out of the treadmill of general practice once they get into it.

It is revealing and somewhat disturbing to read one internist's conception of the personal qualifications which are essential for the specialty of surgery or of internal medicine. While scarcely my conception of the situation, the following words of Dr. James Howard Means[12] are of interest:

> "The personality traits and aptitudes that go to making the good physician differ from those that are needed in the make-up of the good surgeon. The surgeon performs in the lime-light. He is the virtuoso of medicine. His professional work consists to a considerable extent in dealing with crises. At least to the patient the surgical operation is a crisis. The surgeon, who enters and often leaves the patient's life at this time of crisis, in a sense is always on the spot. He must make vital decisions with great rapidity. He must know his way around inside the human body with utter accuracy, certainty and confidence. He must be a robust, resilient, psychologically extroverted sort of person. If he did not have such qualities he could not take what the surgeon has to take.
>
> "The function of the physician is quite different. He is less concerned, at least if he is of the category that I have called 'generalist,' with crises than with the sustained care of patients, keeping them well if he can, or trying to restore them to health if they become sick. He applies any sort of treatment that he is qualified to give and calls in specialists when skills beyond his competence are indicated. The qualities required to make a good physician are understanding, insight, purposeful sympathy, responsibleness and patience. Also, his personality must be one to inspire confidence. He is not on the spot as the surgeon is, and can more readily admit error without losing either face or patient, provided the patient has trust in him. His concern is with the whole patient. He is indeed the personal physician.

"The specialist occupies an intermediate position between the physician and the surgeon in the sense in which I have used these terms. Often, he retains charge of patients for long periods, but he is only taking care of a part of them. The difference, as I see it, between the three categories of practitioners of medicine that I have mentioned is that the surgeon is interested primarily in the operation and the specialist in the disease, but the nonspecialized physician or generalist is interested primarily in the person."

Needless to say, there are pitfalls for the individual who has not experienced a surgical career but who nonetheless presumes to define the qualifications for a surgeon.

At the 73rd meeting of the American Surgical Association in Los Angeles in April 1953, Dr. Frederick A. Coller reported that of the 201,277 physicians in the United States on July 1, 1949, 27.3 per cent (54,891) were full-time specialists and 11.4 per cent (22,-976) were part-time specialists.

The American Medical Association[13] gives the following figures for full-time specialists in 1938, 1949 and 1956, respectively:

SPECIALTY (full time)	NUMBER OF SPECIALISTS		
	1938	1949	1956
Internal medicine	5,688	12,079	16,321
Surgery	5,397	10,363	12,593
Obstetrics and Gynecology	2,227	5,267	7,198
Psychiatry and Neurology	2,154	4,917	7,048
Pediatrics	2,205	4,480	6,567
Ophthalmology, Otology, Laryngology and Rhinology or Otology, Laryngology and Rhinology	5,860	6,753	5,970
Roentgenology and Radiology	1,472	3,038	4,249
Ophthalmology	1,451	2,849	3,694
Orthopedics	984	2,109	3,083
Urology	1,643	2,274	2,746

Figures on certification by the various boards of medical specialties for 1954 are shown in table 1.

The American Surgical Association[14] has stated that a "central authority for certification of surgeons and surgical specialists is needed in which all present and future Boards should be dissolved. Two ranks of certification are suggested."

In an article entitled "The M.D.'s Are Off Their Pedestal," in Fortune Magazine for February 1954, the following figures are given:

PROFESSIONAL FIELD	AVERAGE NET INCOME	AVERAGE HOURS WORK PER WEEK
General Practice	$ 9,561	61
Surgery	17,500	59
Obstetrics and Gynecology	17,000	61
Urology	16,000	55
Orthopedics	19,000	59

The wide ramifications of present-day medical knowledge make specialization a necessity, and it is certainly here to stay. However, specialization is not an unmixed blessing. The Committee on Graduate Surgical Education of the American Surgical Association[14] has warned "against the disintegrating influence of the ever increasing trend toward specialization."

One still hears the remark: "You doctors make me tired! Always sending us around to specialists. Why can't we have the good, old-fashioned family doctor, who took care of everybody and everything at a much more reasonable fee?" The answer which I have found most effective and understandable is: "Why don't you go down to your gas station and tell the men to build you a good, honest automobile from the bottom up, with no specialization frills, no assembly line where one workman just knows how to put on a wheel and another just how to fasten on the gasoline tank." Most people are impressed and even silenced by this argument, despite the fact that, to my mind, it is open to grave criticism. Coordinating a General Motors or Ford assembly line are men of top intelligence —commanding generals, whose education and career qualify them to appraise the relative importance of each of the many component elements in a construction campaign. In the field of medicine, however, there are no exact counterparts to these commanding generals. Nominally the family doctor, who lacks the specialists' experience or training, is the one to evaluate the need of a specialist's services and to choose the specialist himself. Furthermore, every specialist, who corresponds to a highly trained worker on the assembly line, considers himself to be the outstandingly important element in each case, but he lacks the broad perspective and appreciation of the significance and relative importance of the other fields. The situation is much like that in the fable of the blind man who attempted to describe an elephant.

I regard as of utmost importance the impending development in medicine of a means of efficiently and intelligently coordinating

Table 1. *Approved Examining Boards in Medical Specialties**

KEY NO.	NAME OF BOARD	YEAR OF ACTIVATION	TOTAL CERTIFICATES AWARDED TO	
			JULY 1, 1953	JUNE 30, 1954
1.	American Board of Pediatrics..........	1933	4,529	4,964
2.	American Board of Psychiatry and Neurology.........................	1934	4,646	4,931
3.	American Board of Orthopedic Surgery..	1934	2,207	2,354
4.	American Board of Dermatology and Syphilology......................	1932	1,512	1,603
5.	American Board of Radiology.........	1934	4,341	4,649
6.	American Board of Urology...........	1935	1,809	1,921
7.	American Board of Obstetrics and Gynecology........................	1930	3,908	4,291
8.	American Board of Internal Medicine....	1936	8,404	9,062
9.	American Board of Pathology.........	1936	2,494	2,727
10.	American Board of Ophthalmology.....	1917	3,880	4,051
11.	American Board of Otolaryngology.....	1924	4,964	5,073
12.	American Board of Surgery...........	1937	6,158	6,817
13.	American Board of Anesthesiology......	1937	1,023	1,185
14.	American Board of Plastic Surgery......	1937	275	313
15.	American Board of Neurological Surgery.	1940	488	553
16.	American Board of Physical Medicine and Rehabilitation.................	1947	239	240
17.	American Board of Preventive Medicine..	1948	1,068	1,255
18.	American Board of Proctology.........	1949	144	165
	(An Affiliate of the American Board of Surgery).....................	1948	397†	465†
	Totals.....................................		52,486	56,619

* Journal of the American Medical Association *156:*505, 1954.
† Included in totals of American Board of Surgery.

the various specialties. Since enough all-wise individuals to meet the urgent need may never be developed, it may eventually be necessary to have an executive committee type of group, similar to the committees which make high policy decisions in business corporations and banks. Perhaps it would not be too fanciful to suggest that such a coordinator or committee would be somewhat comparable to the conductor of a symphony orchestra. Certainly without the conductor, there might be a tendency for each musician, consciously or unconsciously, to make his part of a symphonic number the most important or most audible. Certainly we are obliged to admit that it is now impossible for the family doctor or general practitioner to become skilled in all the branches of all the specialties.

In his presidential address before the American Surgical Society in 1954, Dr. Howard C. Naffziger[15] said:

"Recently there has been among our medical students a desire to go into general practice. This is a result of the advice they have received. The public regret over the passing of the family doctor and advisor is understandable. The lack of guidance of the individual patient by the specialist if the ailment is not in his line is a common experience, and the poor patient is left at sea. There has been an understandable reaction against such an attitude on the part of the public and by our general practitioners against the emphasis on specialization.

"Nevertheless, there has never been a time when there is less need for general practitioners than today. With the growth of our country, the population has become more and more condensed. Sparsely settled areas are less frequent. With our roads and rapid transportation, medical centers with various specialties represented can supply a far higher level of care than can be given by an equal number of general practitioners. Most often the internist will be the family advisor, because of the greater frequency of ailments of short duration.

"Our need in this country at the present time is for more specialists grouped in centers wherever the population is sufficient to support several doctors. This would make for a higher level of service. The need for general practitioners is diminishing, and the trend of our medical students towards general practice is unfortunate and short-sighted. I believe it will be short lived."

Assuredly, the general practitioner is still indispensable. Spencer[16] wisely observes:

"The physician who chooses to enter the general practice of medicine in a community far removed from hospitals and association with trained surgeons must face and solve problems which do not confront the general practitioner in the city. These problems will involve major injuries. In the city he might be criticized for attempting the care of some of these cases. In a remote area he may open himself to criticism if he does not care for them. There are still communities where kitchen-table surgery is not only justified but imperative. . . . There is probably no field of medicine in which the patient is so completely at the mercy of the doctor as he is in the surgery of trauma."

While the present high degree of specialization in the medical

14

profession has brought great benefit to the patient, since greater skill and learning are brought to bear upon his particular difficulty, it is certainly not faultless. Often a patient is irked when he is obliged to see three or four specialists before a diagnosis is made. The family physician may require the opinion of the gynecologist, the proctologist, the urologist or the allergist or all of them or others. This inevitably makes the cost to the patient higher unless he goes to a clinic where one fee covers all specialists' services. Without question, in the long run an accurate diagnosis and good treatment are the most economical.

The internist has a difficult role to play. On the one hand, he wants to be identified as a specialist in internal medicine, as evidenced by his certificate from the Board of Internal Medicine, with a reputation for advanced knowledge and skill in that specialty. On the other hand, at present he is often the first physician the patient sees and thus, becoming the confidant and family physician, falls into the role of the presumably wise commanding general, who guides in the choice of specialists but wants to feel, in a sense, the patient's continued dependence. He thus becomes a "chameleon"—both an erudite specialist and a "good, old-fashioned" family physician.

The specialist in other branches likewise has certain pitfalls to guard against. He must fight two perils: one, the danger of increasingly assigning more importance to his specialty *per se* than to the over-all patient picture, and, two, the danger of becoming too impersonal in his relationship with patients. He must constantly guard against a narrowing mental outlook by reading about other branches of medicine, by attending general medical meetings and by discussing problems with his colleagues. He will need to reconcile himself to the indubitable fact that the doctor who takes care of Johnny's broken arm will be much more closely known and warmly regarded than the highly skilled man who resects a grandfather's colon or a grandmother's brain tumor. Finally, he must be consistently courageous in differing with the referring doctors when necessary, even at the cost of losing their referred work. On one occasion I declined to remove what I considered to be a normal gallbladder and told the patient so; and that was the last case that his physician ever referred to me.

At present, if a young man has decided to become a specialist, and, what is more difficult, has decided in which particular specialty his interests chiefly lie, he will have to take steps to find and apply for a suitable residency, beginning at the completion of his internship. Preferably, such a residency is for three or four years' duration.

Certification is difficult to obtain. For full details of the rules and requirements, the candidate writes to the secretary of the particular board in which he is interested.[17] Before being permitted to apply for the examinations for certification by the American Board of Surgery, the "Group I" candidate will have to give evidence of:

> "Completion of a graded residency in surgery of at least four years in an institution or institutions acceptable to the board and approved for four years of training by the conference committee on graduate training in surgery. The final year of the program must have been spent in the capacity of senior or chief resident in surgery."

The Board of Surgery provides a second method (Group II) of becoming eligible for examination. It states:

> "Completion of a graded residency in surgery of at least three years in an institution or institutions acceptable to the board and approved for three years of training by the conference committee on graduate training in surgery. The final year must have been spent in the capacity of senior or chief resident in surgery.
> "Credit will be granted for surgical internship to a candidate who has completed one other year of acceptable internship when the surgical internship is part of a graded residency approved for three years by the conference committee.
> "Two additional years of training beyond the three years of residency to complete a total of five are necessary to meet the requirements for examination. These may have been spent (a) in practice limited to surgery carried out under acceptable supervision, (b) in the study of surgery and the basic sciences in an approved graduate school of medicine (no more than one year's credit is granted for work in basic sciences), and (c) in surgical training acceptable to the board in the federal services."
> "Note: In both Group I and Group II, the supervising surgeon must vouch for the candidate's integrity, surgical judgment and technical skill. Sufficient operative work performed independently under supervision to fortify residency training must be attested to by a statement submitted to the board at the time the candidate makes application."

The examinations are in two parts—the first is written and the second is oral and practical. The fee for examination is $150. On April 11, 1956, Dr. John Stewart, chairman of the committee on the American Board of Surgery of the American Surgical Association, reported to that association, in part, as follows:

"During the calendar year, 1955, 816 candidates took the Part I examination of the American Board of Surgery, and of these 633 passed and 183 failed, a failure rate of 22.4%. During the same period 983 candidates took the Part II examination and of these 653 passed and were certified, the failure rate being 33.5%. From the founding of the Board in 1937 to the end of 1955, 6,545 have been certified by examination and the over-all failure rate in the Part II examination has been 29.4%. Occasionally candidates have passed the Part II examination after the second, or even the third, try. If we add to the candidates certified by examination those admitted to certification in the founders group, who number 1,152, the total number of diplomates up to December 31, 1955, was 7,697."

Failure to be certified does not mean that the doctor cannot practice surgery, but it is a serious blow to his chances, since hospital staffs cannot disregard a failure to be certified. Generally speaking, a hospital staff will not exclude a man because he has failed to obtain specialty certification, but nonetheless his chances of full staff membership are greatly improved if he does become certified. The Board states its position as follows:

"The American Board of Surgery has never been concerned with measures that might gain special privileges or recognition for its diplomates in the practice of surgery. *It is neither the intent nor has it been the purpose of the board to define requirement for membership on the staffs of hospitals.* The prime object of the board is to pass judgment on the education and training of broadly competent and responsible surgeons, not who shall or shall not perform surgical operations. The board specifically disclaims interest in or recognition of differential emoluments that may be based on certification."

Residencies are of many grades of desirability, and naturally an ideal surgical residency is visualized differently by different persons. To my mind, it should include a first year in the department of pathology under the guidance and instruction of a first-rate pathologist. During this period the resident should perform as many postmortem examinations as possible and should become skilled in the diagnosis of cases by means of microscopic sections, both frozen and paraffin. He should examine and describe as many as possible of the fresh specimens brought daily from the operating room. He should investigate some special subject with the view of preparing a thesis or similar publication. He should learn to speak before hospital conferences so that he can present a subject briefly, clearly and in an interesting manner.

The resident's last two or three years should be devoted exclusively to surgical work, with a program of increasing responsibility. He should be first assistant in all of the more serious operations, and, gradually, as he demonstrates his competency, he should be permitted to perform operations of increasing difficulty. He should supervise and instruct the surgical interns. He should at all times be fully aware of the condition of the most seriously ill patients in the hospital and should be available to give help in serious cases in the accident room.

Oliver Cope[18] notes that the average age at the time of completion of a residency is 30.5 years and says: "Means must be found as medical knowledge advances to avoid further lengthening of the undergraduate medical curriculum. . . . There is much to recommend the teaching of medicine and surgery as a single discipline." McKittrick[19] says:

> "Probably the most difficult specialty in which to develop a successful practice is that of major surgery. . . . It is not easy for the young surgeon, who may have spent five or six years after graduation preparing to practice the specialty of his choice, to make the necessary adjustment from the protected life of a resident surgeon to the hazards and trials associated with a competitive practice. Formerly everything possible was done to help him; now every possible resistance may be put in his way. . . . These young men know what they are capable of doing. They do not realize that neither the public nor the potential referring physician shares this knowledge, and that until they have become known locally and are able to win the confidence and respect of the local community, the opportunities for them to demonstrate their ability will be infrequent."

CHAPTER II

Choice of Location;
Hospital and Society
Memberships

GENERALLY speaking, there are three broad classifications of possible locations for a surgeon: (1) a small town, of 5,000 to 10,000 population, with its surrounding rural community; (2) a medium-sized city, with a population of 100,000 to 300,000; and (3) a large city with medical schools and affiliated hospitals.

A surgeon cannot locate in a community which does not have a satisfactory hospital. I have seen a splendidly equipped, modern hospital in a town of 3,500 people. Often such a hospital will have no interns, and no training school for nurses, being dependent in the latter department upon salaried graduate nurses. The surgeon usually must depend upon other physicians to help him in operations. The lack of a salaried, full-time pathologist is a great disadvantage, but if biopsy tissues and surgical specimens are sent to the state laboratory or to a private laboratory in a large city, this deficiency can be partly overcome. However, the amount of diagnostic laboratory work is definitely limited.

The surgeon will have to make more house calls and do more work in his office and in patients' homes. His "doctor bag" will be of everyday practical use, and its contents will have to be carefully considered. He will have to attend to all classes of injury, including those of greatest severity and complexity, such as a ruptured spleen and multiple compound fractures. He will have to operate in emergency cases, such as perforated ulcer, acute appendicitis and ruptured ectopic pregnancy, but he will find that many patients requiring elective surgery, such as gallstone and cancer operations, must be sent to a larger town or city. Severe pressure will be put upon him to split fees; in fact the pressure may be so severe that he will have to leave the community to avoid surrendering to it. The important measures which the profession is taking to eradicate fee-splitting will be discussed in a later section.

In a small town the living costs will probably be considerably less than elsewhere. However, the social life may be intense and demanding, and it is almost impossible for one to be independent in this regard. Failure to participate actively in the social merry-go-round may be regarded as snobbishness and may lead to ostracism, with resultant possible loss of practice. In a large city, one's social and intellectual activities can be much more a matter of personal choice.

The imponderable or spiritual rewards, that is, the genuine gratitude and loyalty of one's patients, bring the highest satisfaction and may suffice for a young surgeon's wants. However, if he wishes to become proficient in increasingly difficult operations, to enhance his prestige by means of publications and to enrich his knowledge by stimulating professional contacts, a small community usually raises an insuperable barrier. By force of financial pressure a young surgeon may settle in such a community with the firm intention of going elsewhere when he has accumulated a little financial reserve. But things seldom work out this way, and it takes increasing courage with each passing year to sever ties and make a big change. Security for himself and for his family looms larger than possible greater opportunities in strange new fields. Only an exceptional man can lift himself out of a well-established practice.

The medium-sized city, with a population of 100,000 to 300,000, has much to offer a young surgeon. He can be assured of several first-class hospitals, with competent staffs and with standards approved by the Joint Commission on the Accreditation of Hospitals. He will probably be able to confine his work to the specialty of his choice. The staff meetings of the hospital and of the various medical societies of the city will be vigorous and stimulating. The assistance of a pathology department and of clinical laboratories will be on a high plane. The young surgeon may be able to become an assistant to a distinguished older surgeon, who will be his mentor and will stand back of him as he undertakes operations of increasing magnitude. There may be opportunity to become affiliated with a successful and properly operated group or clinic.

Generally speaking, in a medium-sized city the young surgeon's children will attend better schools. A much wider circle of acquaintances will be available for the entire family from which to select real friends, and these valued friendships can be cultivated with less risk of appearing snobbish or exclusive. Should the surgeon be interested in and have time for participation in civic affairs, these activities may be more readily pursued than in a large city.

For ultimate advancement and development, a large city—and this includes the immediate suburbs—offers the most for the young surgeon. However, large cities are most impersonal, and the acquisition of a practice by the fundamental route of the satisfied patient is much slower than in a small city or a rural community. At first the young surgeon's practice seldom is sufficient to use up all his time and energy. These are the years when earnest work in the medical school, without pay, is most rewarding and necessary and when supplementary salaried, part-time (!) positions must be sought to help provide an income.

If a young surgeon has a reasonably satisfactory record, appointment to the medical school faculty should be obtained without difficulty. An appointment below the professorial rank may be made by the head of a department without consultation with other faculty members. The beginning rank is usually that of "instructor," and the first work assigned is usually that of helping to teach the third year students in the surgical outpatient department. If the instructor's work is satisfactory, he may be promoted and become an "assistant" and then an "associate" and given charge of some classwork. Beyond the grade of "associate" come the grades of "assistant professor," "associate professor" and (full) "professor," all of which are granted only upon recommendation of an appropriate committee, followed by favorable action by the medical council.

During these early years in a large city the young surgeon will have the opportunity and usually the time to initiate or to participate in some research work. Older men in the medical school are always needing the help of younger men to assist in some research project. For a young surgeon to engage in these projects is rewarding, as he will become proficient in the use of some of the techniques of investigation, e.g., in animal surgery, bacteriological studies and chemical studies.

However, the young surgeon must not be content for too long to accept a subordinate role; soon he must originate and test an idea of his own. Moreover, at the outset he must face head-on the concept that, despite the intense efforts of medical school departments to increase the mere quantity of research publications, *not everyone* is qualified to engage in research. Truly dedicated research workers are relatively few and far between and should be well cared for, protected and salaried by medical schools, not being obliged to engage in private practice. As I have stated earlier, somewhat ironically, perhaps some day we shall have an American Board of Research, which will decide who is competent enough and deserves to be permitted to engage in research work. This is quite at variance with the present plan, which tends to take it for granted that every medical student is a potential research worker, or at least should be considered so until proved incompetent, regardless of the waste of his time and energy.

Often, the most valuable type of investigation is the careful study of groups of cases in an effort to evaluate accurately a method of treatment. Henry K. Beecher[20] has wisely said:

> "It is just possible, however, that there is still a place in clinical investigation for the great idea preserved, protected, and developed with no more physical tools than the notebook and pencil . . . even the newest investigator does not seem to think he can function unless he has one or more complex (and expensive) instruments. The whole crazy, upside-down situation was illustrated the other day in a short letter that said, 'Dear Doctor, I have bought an oximeter. Will you suggest a research problem to use it on?' "

In his presidential address before the American College of Surgeons Elkin[21] noted that:

> ". . . mankind cries out for light and still more light. That light can be shed by men who do not have elaborate laboratory facilities at their command. When Mackenzie began the research that ultimately made him the greatest heart specialist of his time, it was because a young woman with a cardiac condition had died in childbirth. He had not expected her to die. Like Hippocrates, Jenner, Bright, Addison, the Hunters, Colles, and a host of others, he had no x-rays, no pathologic

laboratories, and not much in the way of diagnostic facilities except what he created himself. He was, he said, under the prevalent belief that medical research could only be undertaken in a laboratory, or, at least, in a hospital with all the appurtenances. So, when he began, he merely sought to find out something about the nature of patients' complaints. That same road is still open."

In his colorful article entitled "Please Call a Doctor," James H. Spencer[16] says:

"Just as there are general practitioners who long for opportunities to take things out of the human body and miss their chances to put things back where they belong, so there are surgeons who dream of being pioneers in the cutting art and in the stupor of their dreams sleep away their chances of saving more lives and limbs than they would ever save by operations which make the front pages of newspapers. The departments of research are combing the human body for new areas of attack. . . . I am not at all sure but what I am safer riding in my high-powered car or playing with my machine tools than I would be to enter a university hospital with high blood pressure, cirrhosis of the liver or even cold feet."

Publication of the report of a rare case, after a truly intensive search of the world's literature, is always useful and commendable. The study of groups of similar cases in hospital record rooms has been given a death blow, or at least has been made immeasurably more difficult, by the introduction of microfilming of records. No longer is it possible to run through a pile of charts and sift out one comparable item at a time.

In a large city many opportunities can be found for earning money professionally outside of private practice. The commonest of these is the position as physician on duty in a large plant or industry. Here the young surgeon makes routine physical examinations and cares for employees who have accidents and illnesses. Most of these positions are full-time, but it is almost mandatory for the young surgeon to find one that is part-time; otherwise he will be unable to develop his private practice or engage in medical school activities. Life insurance examination is another source of revenue. Also there are salaried positions in student health activities and in various night clinics.

Membership in an established group, association or partnership is often possible and, if the conditions are proper, is usually desirable.[22] Many types of groups are found, and much has been written about them. The American Association of Medical Clinics (established in 1949) has in its by-laws the following provisions concerning eligibility for full membership:

"Any group of seven or more full-time physicians maintaining a private organization for the purposes of providing general medical care of high quality . . . shall be eligible for membership. Such group or clinic shall have on its full-time staff at least five physicians in different major specialties, two of which specialties shall be internal medicine and general surgery. Such group shall maintain a separate building or suite of offices for the conduct of its practice."

Jordan,[23] in an article adapted from a chapter entitled "Group Practice" from his book, *The Physician, His Business and His Practice,* says:

"There are several methods by which group-practice clinics may be classified—by size, by nature of services rendered and by internal structure and organization. Some are large, with physician staffs ranging into hundreds. Others are small partnerships of three or four men. . . . Most groups consist of practitioners who have banded together into private organizations. In some, physicians connected with a hospital or medical school have joined in what is surely one kind of group practice. Some groups are sponsored by consumers and are usually known by the name of health co-operatives. In a few cases the establishment of prepaid programs has led to the development of medical groups designed to care for the patients enrolled under such insurance plans. In some groups the physicians are all in one specialty, such as radiology, internal medicine, or dermatology. All the physicians in some clinics are specialists in various fields; in others physicians in general practice play an important part, and in still others the groups are composed exclusively of general practitioners. . . . Except in a few states a corporation cannot practice medicine. For this reason the vast majority of group-practice clinics are organized as partnerships. Again, the variation in the details of agreement is remarkable. Some consist of two or three original partner founders, the other physicians in the group serving as employees of the partnership. More often, a definite pattern of entry into the partnership is available for physicians joining the group. A trial period averaging two or three years before admission to the partnership is common, but not invariable. Sometimes a junior partnership has been established as a step preceding the attainment of full partnership status. Another aspect of most partnerships that should be mentioned is that the more experienced groups have generally found it impracticable to continue indefinitely an equal division of income among the partners or even to weigh the influence of all partners in the affairs of the group exactly alike. Consequently many devices have been adopted to make the partnership structure fit into a smoothly functioning operation. If a corporation could legally practice medicine it would have numerous advantages over the partnership, especially for the groups of larger size. Since it usually cannot, however, a 'new' form of group practice has begun to develop. This is an organization that can be described briefly as an unincorporated association of physicians. This structure permits all the physicians in the group to be on a salary established by an elected board of trustees or governors, and therefore it can be operated in much the same manner as a corporation. . . . As a long-term proposition . . . equal division of net earnings is probably impracticable."

Jordan describes the many different schemes to divide the group's income and concludes: "Certainly, the physicians in a group should not expect perfection from any plan to divide their income, but should attempt to make it work as well as possible." He further states that the National Association of Clinic Managers, organized in 1926, "has rendered the medical profession great service in gathering information concerning appropriate business methods and in standardizing certain types of business procedures." The American Association of Medical Clinics is more concerned with the professional aspects and also maintains a placement service "to physicians desiring to associate themselves with a group practice and to group-practice clinics that desire additional professional personnel." In 1954 the association estimated that 7,000 doctors in the United States are in group practice.

Much can be said in favor of the general plan of group practice. Men of different interests and different specialties can become associated economically in one building and share the expenses of rent, services and the like. Moreover, the many informal exchanges of opinions are educational and stimulating, being conducive both to the patient's interest and to the physician's professional education. The group idea generally appeals to and attracts patients. A young man who becomes associated with a fine group will immediately be busy seeing many patients and earning money and will be afforded many opportunities for professional discussion. His life is usually much more congenial and stimulating than when he starts as a "lone wolf." Burrows,[24] writing in 1925, was skeptical of clinics and warned of the "fallacy of collective responsibility. . . . Medicine is an art, and no work of art can reach a high level when it is the product of a group of individuals, each of whom has a controlling interest. . . . Who will suppose that a first-class portrait could be produced by a congery of artists? . . . The specialists are useful, are essential. But in the last arbitrament the clinician must remain supreme." Excellent guides for the young physician for solving some of the problems of practice have been written by Joseph Garland[25] and George E. Hall.[26]

Admittedly, some groups which were started with enthusiasm have failed, the chief cause of failure being an unjust and improper organizational plan. The fundamental plan in setting up a successful group must have two indispensable cornerstones. First, each member of the group must receive financial return in exact proportion to his earnings for the group. A useful method is to have an annual computation of the percentage of the total group's receipts which each man has contributed and let that be his percentage of income after expenses. Properly he may take vacations during the year totaling but usually not over three months, since his diminished contribution to the receipts would be reflected in his next year's percentage. It may be proper that he share equally in some joint expenses, such as reception room rent, or at a similar percentage. The second cornerstone to success is the fixed principle that no member of the group is obliged to refer a patient for special treatment only to some other member of the group. He may refer the patient to some member of the group if he feels that that physician is competent to do the work and is acceptable to the patient. However, it must be strictly understood by all the members of the group that such referrals are entirely optional.

A young surgeon who becomes associated with a group is usually taken on a probationary basis, with an agreement which may be renewed from year to year. He may be on a straight salary or on a salary plus a bonus which is dependent upon the amount that his receipts exceed his salary. The "probationer" usually has no rent, telephone or office supply expenses. In the great clinics, such as the Mayo Clinic, the Lahey Clinic and the Crile Clinic, each doctor is in the fortunate position of being on a straight salary. His daily work does not have a piecemeal relationship to his remuneration, but of course the general excellence of his work is reflected in his salary. Jordan[27] has recently contributed an excellent discussion on the business side of group practice.

Another plan is for a young surgeon to become associated as a salaried assistant to an older surgeon. This is a common and usually mutually profitable arrangement. The junior surgeon relieves the senior of many time-taking tasks, such as evening rounds at the hospital and house calls, helps in doing dressings in the office and hospital and in preparing medical papers and, where a residency system is not involved, assists in operations. The senior, or preceptor, teaches the younger man all he knows of surgery, backs him up in his first operations, introduces him to patients and teaches him by example how to talk to them, helps him become a member of various surgical societies and stimulates him to study and to contribute to the surgical literature.

Almost invariably such an association must of necessity terminate after a variable interval of time. As the junior surgeon becomes more proficient and if he is made of the right stuff, he naturally yearns to accept greater responsibility and begins to chafe at being an assistant. In time he either tumbles out of the nest on his own or is crowded out. Meanwhile, the senior surgeon has felt increasingly that it is inappropriate to call upon the younger man for the tasks of an assistant. Inevitably some patients will show a preference for the junior surgeon, a circumstance which tends to inflate the junior and to pain the senior. Just before this time arrives, it is best for the junior's future and for development of his surgical stature to go out on his own, and it will be better for the senior to have a new and younger assistant. Sometimes the problem is solved by having the junior and senior form a partnership and acquire a third man as an assistant to both of them. Such an arrangement is feasible only if the increase in operative work is such as to keep all three busy.

The matter of hospital staff membership has already been discussed, and all the observations apply with regard to a large city hospital. However, in a large city the hospital usually is affiliated with a medical school and is a "teaching hospital," the staff members accepting the additional responsibility of instructing interns, residents, clerks and third and fourth year medical students. No physician can become a member of the staff of a teaching hospital unless he is a member of the faculty of the medical school. A discussion of the manner of instruction in a hospital will be taken up later.

The subject of socialized medicine is usually discussed intemperately. However, it is the duty of all medical men to be thoroughly informed as to its implication and the current trends toward it. Dr. Means[22] says: "The impulse to reform in medical public affairs comes usually from without, and resistance to it from within the majority fold of organized medicine. . . . It is only under the lash of public opinion that organized medicine makes any social progress."

Walton H. Hamilton,[28] a distinguished law professor at Yale, once said while dissenting from the 1932 report of the majority of the Committee on American Medicine:

> "If we are to make the most of our human resources, for work and for life, it is necessary that our facilities for health shall be just as available for all who need them as are the schools and the churches. Nor should the matter of a membership in a health service be left to the free choice of the individual. The 'reasonable man' of our ancestors, who was prudent and provident and would always seek his own best advantage, now lives only as a fiction."

I am not certain that competition results in the degree of progress in medicine that it does in automotive engineering, electronics and the airplane industry. In the latter fields the consumer is better qualified to judge the products than is the patient with regard to the field of medicine.

When a young surgeon is ready to start his own practice, he must decide on the locality in which he wishes to work and live. In many instances this problem has been settled by associations made in medical school or during his internship or residency. Since localities differ greatly, many different motives must be considered in making a decision. However, no matter what choice is made, complete satisfaction is seldom achieved. In fact, the surgeon may have to change to another locality, but, by and large, this is to be avoided, if possible. A man who has spent his life in a large city may believe that he would have been happier in a small town or rural community, where he would be closer to his friends and patients, closer to nature, and, at least in his conception of it, where the pace would have been slower, with more time spent with his family and more time for recreation. Likewise, the man in a rural community or small town, even after a long and successful career, may imagine that if he had only stayed in a large city the stimulating effects of a medical school and large hospital associations would have made him more progressive and more alert to medical progress. Fortunately, some surgeons find city life abhorrent, while others find it fascinating and essential to their happiness.

A compromise is chosen by some surgeons by settling in the suburb of a large city, a solution which has many advantages. He can drive daily, if necessary, to a medical school for teaching or research work, he can be on the staff of a "teaching hospital" which is affiliated with the medical school, and he can attend important surgical society meetings more readily than if he lived in a rural community. Moreover, while he still takes care of charity patients, either at a medical school or at a hospital, his practice will have a larger proportion of families who live in the suburbs because they find better schools for their children, more healthful surroundings and more congenial friends. Such families are usually quick to consult a physician and may be more appreciative of his services.

The young surgeon may give some thought to finding a locality where there is a dearth of doctors. However, this factor should not be stressed too heavily, as the best place to find work is where there are many doctors, since that is where the demand for surgical care is greatest. Of course the newcomer must meet the competition from others by rendering his best services.

The chief stimulus for building up a successful practice comes from satisfied, grateful patients. This is why competition rather than "socialized" or state medicine probably is most advantageous for the patients. Spencer[16] observes:

> "For the young physician who by force of circumstances needs to make for himself a reputation as soon as possible, I would suggest two things. First, deliver some babies. If you don't interfere too much with nature, your fame will grow and spread. Then don't miss an opportunity to stop the pain, soothe the nerves and restore normal function in as many accidents as possible. The young mothers and the injured citizens will sing your praises and oftentimes pay your bill."

In selecting a locality, a young doctor must consider his professional career first, for if his career is successful, his family will usually prosper. But when he must make a choice between several more or less equal opportunities, a consideration of the welfare and happiness of his wife and children becomes more vital.

As soon as a young surgeon has chosen his locality, he must become a staff member of a hospital of the highest possible quality. Such hospitals are fully accredited by the Joint Commission on Accreditation (JCAH). This commission was formed on January 1, 1953, and is the outgrowth of the hospital-inspection program conducted by the American College of Surgeons for the last thirty-five years. The JCAH now is composed of representatives of the American College of Surgeons, the American College of Physicians, the American Hospital Association, the American Medical Association and the Canadian Medical Association. Each accredited hospital has a staff that is properly organized, somewhat after the manner prescribed by the American College of Surgeons standards. Regular staff meetings are held, a president is elected annually and a number of active committees handle the multiplicity of staff administrative duties, such as the selection of interns and the supervision of records, library, outpatient department, pharmacy and the like. The various branches and departments of the hospital hold their periodic meetings for the review and discussion of professional subjects. The entire staff attend weekly professional meetings, guided preferably by the department of pathology. The hospital has a close liaison between the board of directors, the administrator or superintendent, and the medical staff—a liaison which is usually most effective if the governing group is small and meets frequently to consider matters of over-all policy and to make decisions. Such a group usually includes the chairmen of the various departments and the current president of the staff. The chairmen may be appointed by the board or elected by the staff, either for an indefinite or for a definite term. If the latter, a period of not less than three years is desirable.

It is important that the staff members feel that their representatives on the executive committee really represent them and keep them informed. For purely professional matters, a smaller committee, consisting of department heads and the administrator, act on such matters as admission to the staff and instruction of interns. The staff has a constitution and by-laws which have been approved by both the staff and the board of directors of the hospital.

One of the most important factors in an appraisal of a hospital's professional standing is the percentage of postmortem examinations relative to the total number of hospital deaths. Generally speaking, the higher the percentage of postmortem examinations, the higher the quality of professional care and standards. A necropsy rate of 75 to 80 per cent warrants a high rating. Below 50 per cent is distinctly low grade. A young surgeon before applying for hospital staff privileges should investigate the statistics in this regard, as well as the organization of the staff and the standing and careers of its members. Such information can be obtained from the American College of Surgeons and the American Medical Association.

An applicant cannot expect acceptance on a fine hospital staff unless he has a record of intelligence and energy. If he is "board-certified," his chances are vastly better. He may be made a member of a probationary group for three to five years; after which time, if he has not made the expected progress, he will be dropped. In a so-called "closed" hospital, only physicians on the staff may admit patients to the hospital, but most hospitals have a group called the "courtesy staff," who may admit patients but who have no voice in staff deliberations. Both regular and courtesy staff appointments are made by the hospital board upon recommendation of the executive committee of the staff, usually on an annual basis. Once accepted, the young surgeon should work hard at the various tasks assigned to him, some of which will not be stimulating, such as work on the records committee or the library committee, but all medical leaders have risen via these humble duties.

If the young surgeon settles in a city having a medical school, it is to his advantage to apply for a teaching position. In fact, as previously stated, faculty membership is a prerequisite when applying for staff membership in a "teaching hospital," that is, a hospital affiliated with a medical school. Membership on a medical school faculty is of great value to the young surgeon, as it brings him into contact with men of high professional standing, it obliges him to study rigorously and keep up to date regarding medical progress, and is a factor leading to admission to special societies. At present these advantages are of such value and the expense of maintaining a medical school are so heavy that young instructors are not paid for their services. It is to be hoped that some way will soon be found to remedy this deficiency, since better instruction would result if competition was keen for teaching positions. While much of the teaching is done on the premises of the medical school, an increasing amount is being done at the affiliated hospitals.

The young surgeon should make every effort to become a fellow in the American College of Surgeons and to win certification by the American Board of Surgery. He should promptly apply for membership in the county medical society, which includes membership in the state medical society and in the American Medical Association. The next step in the ladder of special societies is the surgical society in his city, if it is large enough to have one; for example, the Chicago Surgical Society or the Minneapolis Surgical Society. Usually one does not apply for membership in such a society but must be proposed by three sponsors. If the application is passed by the executive council of the society, the candidate is voted upon at the annual meeting by secret ballot. Needless to say, the executive council has a heavy responsibility in maintaining the high quality of a society's membership, but it should avoid the pitfall of permitting the mere number of papers published by a candidate to be the deciding factor in its deliberations.

Membership in the local surgical society is of extreme importance, perhaps more so than membership in the distinguished and more select national or sectional groups. Take the Chicago Surgical Society for example. Except during the summer months, meetings are held on the first Friday of each month. In the morning are scheduled operations, "dry" clinics and presentations of research work at each of the great Chicago area hospitals and teaching centers in rotation. Many out-of-town men make a habit of attending these instructive morning sessions, which are followed by a luncheon. The evening or "scientific" meeting is preceded by a dinner, a most enjoyable affair at which lasting and valuable friendships are formed. Many a surgical problem is discussed, and by the exchange of experiences with old friends the surgeon continues his education. The formal evening program consists of four or five papers, each followed by a general discussion. Many new pieces of work are presented first before this society, sometimes by a young surgeon who is not as yet a member of the society but "by invitation" of one of the members reports the results of some investigation. This has an important place in the stimulation and encouragement of the younger men, but must not be overdone at the cost of reducing the number of clinical reports presented by the older, leading surgeons. Furthermore, the program committee must not permit the society's forum to be overused as a reward for the many workers who perform a piece of work for an older surgeon. The president, or presiding officer, should encourage free discussion of each paper and should call upon the older men to give their opinions.

The next objectives in the matter of society memberships to be aimed at by the young surgeon are the more exclusive surgical societies, which are not national but are comprised of men from a limited area of the country. Examples of these societies are the Western Surgical Association, the Southern Surgical Association, the Pacific Coast Surgical Association and the Central Surgical Association. These societies usually have an annual three-day or four-day meeting in a large city in the area. The sessions are long and, as many papers are presented, often fatiguing. Since all of the papers can be read later in the published transactions, the chief advantage of attending the meetings is to meet and talk with some of the leaders in surgery.

In the United States the surgical society which is generally considered to carry the most prestige is the American Surgical Association. This great society, sometimes referred to as the "Brahmins," was founded in 1880 by Samuel D. Gross, who became its first president. Among its presidents have been many of the great men in American surgery, including Senn, Warren, Keen, Matas, William and Charles Mayo, J. M. T. Finney, L. L. McArthur, Crile, A. J. Ochsner, D. F. Jones, E. W. Archibald and Evarts Graham. This society, whose active membership is limited to 250, has had a powerful influence in assuring and maintaining the high standards of surgery in this country. Next in importance to the American Surgical Association come the Society of Clinical Surgery and the Society of University Surgeons. In addition, there are numerous more specialized societies, such as the American Association for the Surgery of Trauma, the Society of Neurological Surgeons, the American Urological Association, the American Orthopedic Association, the American Goitre Association and the American Society of Plastic and Reconstructive Surgery. One hundred and seventy-seven American and foreign societies are listed in the American College of Surgeons directory.

Another type of surgical society is the so-called "travel club," composed of a small group of congenial surgical leaders who meet annually in a different medical center, where new work is presented and discussed and a great deal is learned from conversations with old friends over the three to four days of meetings. I am happy to be a member of the Halsted Society, named in honor of William S. Halsted, the illustrious professor of surgery at Johns Hopkins. This club has ninety-three members, twenty-seven of whom are now listed as senior members. Nearly all of the men are professors of surgery, and many are heads of departments in the great medical schools, a highly interesting and stimulating group.

CHAPTER III

Early Surgical Practice

I<small>T</small> <small>IS</small> of utmost importance that the young surgeon make arrangements so that he can always be reached by telephone at any time in the twenty-four hours. I found that my life was much more peaceful if I had a telephone in the dining room, in my den and in practically every other room in the house. Ready accessibility saves not only time but temper, is especially desirable in cases of emergency and is of vital importance when the condition of a hospitalized patient takes an unfavorable turn. The surgeon must resign himself to the fact that he must be readily accessible in any restaurant or theater; for example, in a movie theater he must ask an usher to note where he is sitting so that he can be notified of a telephone call. Years ago, when I used to try to get in some golf, my game was frequently spoiled by having a caddy bicycle out to any part of the course to notify me of an emergency. Sports such as sailing should not be undertaken unless one or two substitute surgeons are available. If a physicians' telephone exchange service is available a surgeon should always subscribe to it. This service includes some such listing in the telephone directory after each doctor's name as this: "If no answer, call DA8–1789." Whenever leaving his home or office, the physician registers with the exchange so that he can be reached quickly if necessary.

Much has been written about doctors' offices and reception rooms, special emphasis being placed on a friendly atmosphere, courteous personnel, including the receptionist, office nurse and bookkeeper, and proper filing of patients' records, which must be kept strictly up to date.

The young surgeon's first patients usually have minor injuries which require prompt attention, such as lacerations, burns and lesser fractures. As there are certain practical considerations which are helpful in the proper care of these conditions, I shall illustrate them in the following section by citing actual examples.

I often tell interns and residents that the most important and instructive cases they are studying will be of value to them throughout their careers. The pertinent facts are stored away in mental pigeonholes, seemingly forgotten, but ready to be called out when needed, even years later. Many cases are noteworthy either because of their professional aspects or because of their social value. Various incidents of my practice that occurred twenty or thirty years ago come to mind as vividly as though they had happened yesterday.

The diagnosis of most fractures is usually self-evident from the history of a recent injury and a painful, immobile, sometimes deformed extremity. No doctor who wishes to be successful in his practice palpates unduly or perhaps at all when a fracture is suspected. If an extremity is painful after an injury, *never* try to save the patient expense by omitting an x-ray examination. Occasionally a patient grumbles when no fracture is found in the x-ray, and complains that unnecessary expense has been entailed, but when an x-ray is not taken immediately and a fracture is later (perhaps elsewhere) discovered, the patient seldom forgives you and may even sue.

The physician is not always as fortunate as I was in a certain case. A woman telephoned me that her little girl had fallen while roller skating and had hurt her wrist. "Do you think you should see it?" she asked. I, not wanting to appear to be trying to "run up business" for myself, and unaware of the pitfall in the situation replied, "No." The next day the mother called me and complained that the child had cried all night, so I insisted on having an x-ray made, which revealed a slight, impacted fracture of the lower end of the radius without displacement. No setting was required, but the child felt somewhat better when the arm was put at rest with a splint and sling. The mother's comment was, "Well, doctor, we certainly were fooled, weren't we!" I saw the same thing happen to another physician, but in his case the patient, an adult, took revenge by continuous malicious gossip and injured the doctor's reputation. About 70 per cent of all malpractice suits are concerned with fractures. Failure to apply a cast or splints properly and to follow the patient carefully for the first few days is rarely condoned.

I have set a "greenstick" fracture without using an anesthetic in a few cases in which a child was courageous and cooperative, but practically always an anesthetic is necessary. To give an anesthetic to an unprepared child, whose stomach is full or at least partly so, takes great skill and is far more dangerous than the laity realize. The doctor is importuned to "give something so he will not feel pain." This, of course, the doctor wants to do and, moreover, must do in order to relax the muscular spasm which otherwise might prevent or at least greatly interfere with the reduction (setting) of the fracture.

Minor lacerations in the case of a very young child with frightened, solicitous, excitable parents may tax the skill, tact, patience and ingenuity of the doctor. As a rule, a child will cooperate better if the parents are not present, or at least are silent and cooperative. The ordeal becomes more severe when a parent reiterates: "Johnny, the doctor will not hurt you!" or "Johnny, be sure to tell the doctor when he hurts you!" Never fear, Johnny will always let you know when it hurts and sometimes when it does not. C. Anderson Aldrich made many sage observations regarding children, but one which sticks in my mind particularly and which I have passed on to many medical students is: "Never ask a child if it hurts." Aldrich, from his rich and wide experience, knew that a child will *always* voluntarily let you know when something hurts and will practically always answer in the affirmative when asked if something hurts, regardless of whether it does or not.

The ability to get close to a child and to win his confidence, trust and cooperation is largely a reflection of what kind of man the doctor is, the sum total of his upbringing, experiences and nature. Some men are magically blessed with the right quality, while others never can develop it. Oversolicitude or a "gushing" voice usually arouses instant suspicion in a child, as past experience has taught him that some malevolent plot is probably associated with that approach and that a preliminary, subtle conspiracy is under way to get him to do something he does not want to do. Certainly a loud voice should not be used. The doctor simply explains what has to be done. He should never say, "I will not hurt you," but, "I will be as careful as I can and will hurt you just as little as possible." Or, "It will not hurt much, and I will tell you just when to expect the worst hurt." By conversing with a child, one can usually distract his attention from his injury and from your treatment of it, but the language used must be what the child understands. Always call him by his first name. Discuss subjects which make sense to him, such as running. "Can you run fast? Can you run as fast as a dog? As fast as an automobile? Do you like ice cream? What is your favorite kind?" Always tell the mother that the child should have more ice cream. "Do you have a dog? What's his name? A cat? An elephant? Have you been to the zoo? Were you scared? Did the elephant bite you?" Sometimes the doctor is rewarded by a loud laugh, in which event he has indeed made progress.

No more difficult ordeal is confronted by the physician (and by all others concerned) than the dressing of a painful wound or the placement of stitches in a frightened child of three or four years attended by his mother in the physician's office. Sometimes the doctor can get the assistance of some one close at hand, but occasionally he must have recourse to the primitive procedure of tightly wrapping the child in a sheet as a restraint. More and more the present-day practitioner has the good fortune of being able to do this work in the accident or emergency room of a nearby hospital, where he has the trained assistance of nurses and usually interns.

Perhaps the most difficult test of the surgeon's finesse, patience, wisdom and skill is an abdominal examination of a child of two or three years. A serious decision depends upon the findings of such an examination, and it is virtually impossible to learn anything if the child is crying. The surgeon's aim is to secure, in his small patient, complete relaxation of the abdomen as a result of the child's dissociation of interest in the examination. Usually the surgeon's introduction to the situation is in the child's room, with the parents visibly grim and anxious to have a decision made quickly and accurately (of course). "Tell us the truth doctor. We can take it." Before the doctor's arrival every child becomes infected by the parents' anxiety, especially in those few homes where the "sagacious" parents say to the child, "If you're not good, I'll call the doctor."

I have found the following technique of value. On entering the room, do not look at the child or pay any particular attention to him. You can almost feel the intensity of the child's appraisal of you. A direct approach to the child, with smiles, honeyed words and blandishments is usually doomed to failure. Instead of looking at the child, become interested in something connected with or in the room: the view from the window, a dog or cat, pictures on the wall, a desk or bookcase, but best of all some toy, particularly a mechanical one. Under no circumstances work the toy successfully; struggle vainly to operate it and, unless a dull-witted parent intercedes, the child will practically always demonstrate how the toy works. The small course of instruction should be prolonged as much as possible, and during this time the child discovers that the doctor has human qualities, at least. If you can casually approach the child's bedside and sit down in a chair, you can then proceed with a more or less man-to-man conversation with him on such sensible topics as running, food and animals, as previously mentioned.

Now comes the time to use a most important maneuver. You must tell "The Bear Story," not in simple narrative form but interrupted by many questions on your part. "I was driving through the Canadian Rockies last summer when what do you think walked right out of the woods?" (Several guesses by the child, we hope.) "It was a bear! A big black bear. And do you know what I did?" "No, what?" "I stopped the car and gave the bear a sandwich. He stood up on his hind legs. You know you can't give a bear half a sandwich, because he will grab for the other half and may hurt you. Then, do you know what I did?" "No, what?" "I took the bear's picture. I have the picture in my pocket. Would you like to see it?" Always the answer is, "Yes." Now, two details are important. First, your hand must be warm. No child will tolerate a cold, clammy hand on his stomach. The fact that you must "feel his stomach to make him better" will by this time become, usually, quite subordinate to the interest in the bear picture. The second detail is that the child must hold the picture *with both his hands,* which further distracts his interest from you and lets you use both your hands, one to lift up the bedcovers a little and the other for palpating gently. While the child is examining the bear picture, you must keep up a running chatter of information and questions about the bear. I have seen a child forget the examination entirely. If at this juncture the mother brightly says, "Now, Johnny, tell the doctor if it hurts!" then the whole campaign may collapse like a house of cards, and you are tempted to tell the mother what you think, which of course would only make matters worse. Meanwhile, you should be palpating with utmost gentleness, always starting in a region which you think will not have any tenderness and last of all reaching the suspected tender part, the right lower quadrant. *Never press hard where you know it will not hurt,* as the child will expect you to press hard where he knows it does hurt and will give a misleading defensive reaction. Often he will beg to keep your bear picture, so be sure to have a few extra copies for that purpose.

One time I operated on a large, strong, intellectual, high-strung Dane, whose wife called him a "Viking." He was courageous and uncomplaining in the painful days after the operation and held himself rigid and tense. In an attempt to divert him, I described the manner in which I told my bear story to children and then showed him the snapshot. This stratagem was very successful as he was genuinely interested. When I found he was interested also in the "Kensington Stone," the stone with Norse characters on it which was found in Minnesota and thought possibly to have been left by the Vikings, I began to register my genuine interest in it. Soon his thoughts were busily engaged in suggesting suitable articles for me to read on the subject. These, in due time, were lent to me, but happily he was then recovered and I no longer needed the story in order to examine him. Apparently I did not show my former interest, for his wife later reported that they had concluded that the Kensington Stone was just another type of "Bear Story."

I have included these details because of their importance. Literally life or death may hang on the result of a successful examination, albeit less so now than in the early days when no antibiotics were available to help when a correct diagnosis could not be made. I shall never forget the instance of a certain frightened, crying four-year-old boy. An older, very distinguished pediatrician had made a diagnosis of acute appendicitis. I was a young man then and had considerable temerity to disagree with my older colleague. Soon another surgeon was called, and he agreed with me. The next day "rose spots" appeared on the child's abdomen, typhoid fever being the correct diagnosis. Had an appendectomy been performed, harm could have resulted.

The human understanding of a physician may be judged by his reply to the frequently posed question of a patient regarding a pain. "Could it be a nerve, doctor?" The wise doctor may justifiably reply, "Yes, there is a strong probability that such is the case. I think you have the right idea." The inexperienced doctor, however, would reply, with perhaps a superior air, "Any one should know that the only way pain is reported is by a nerve. There can be no sensation of pain without involvement of a nerve."

When I began to operate at the Evanston Hospital, I kept constantly in mind the sage advice of my one-time chief, Dr. Albert E. Halstead: "You are a young man. When a patient is in a grave condition and is likely to die, always have senior consultation, even if you feel confident that nothing different can be done. It will save the family worry and will enhance rather than detract from their respect for you." I was somewhat surprised to find that after I had cared for a cook or gardener with great patience, his wealthy employer would engage me for himself and his family later when medical help was needed. A good, safe rule which should be obvious for every young doctor is to treat *each* patient with all the care and skill he can, regardless of the number of patients he has or the financial standing of each patient. Often a small community provides a fine stimulus for a young doctor. His work and degree of patience and his kindliness are observed and discussed minutely there, whereas in the jungles of the big city any brusque action can often be overlooked and a surgeon is more likely to become impersonal and unsympathetic.

One day Dr. Frank W. Blatchford called me to see a shrewd, highly intelligent millionaire who lived in a veritable palace on the lake front. My model T Ford looked ill at ease in the sweeping driveway banked with beds of flowers. From the moment I first heard the patient's name, my heart sank and I quaked in dire foreboding: "Would he recognize me as the idiot who had tried to sell him the idea of a 'noiseless plate'?"

To explain my perturbation, it will be necessary to turn back about two years, to the period when I was spending much time in the John Crerar Library preparing medical articles. I often ate lunch at what was then called the "Automat," where one put coins in a slot to get the plate of food seen through a little glass door. Somehow the clatter and bang of the china on the tables and trays seemed unnecessarily loud and annoying. I dreamed up a "noiseless plate," and the more I thought about it the more practicable it seemed. I drew plans of a plate with special insets over the prominences and with rubber rings to slip over these insets. Such plates could surely be banged around freely without noise. The next thing was to interest someone in my invention, and no one would know better than Mr. X, president of the huge organization dealing with restaurant supplies. It was difficult to get an appointment to see him personally, but finally the day arrived when I was ushered into the great man's office. He listened to me politely but with a definite twinkle in his eye and finally ended the interview by commenting: "I think your best interests would be served by confining your activities to the field of medicine!" Yes, the man of the "noiseless plate" incident was none other than the patient Dr. Blatchford asked me to see.

Fortunately, Mr. X did not recognize me. I examined him carefully, made a diagnosis of a severe attack of acute appendicitis and advised prompt operation. Dr. Edwards, then dean of Northwestern University Medical School, was called into consultation and concurred with my diagnosis. Although the patient had confidence in Dr. Blatchford, who vouched for me, I believe his final decision to let such a young man as I was operate on him was influenced by my stating: "Next to you, Mr. X., I am the person most concerned, since my reputation is at stake because of your prominence." So, I operated on him for a ruptured appendix, and he made an excellent recovery.

I cannot deny that thoughts of the size of the fee I should charge him had flitted through my mind. However, I was really unprepared when one day, as I was completing the dressing, he looked at me sharply and said: "How much are you going to charge me?" He had caught me off balance, and I could not muster the speech I had been trying to formulate. All that I managed to stammer out was a comment to the effect that my fee had to show some relationship to his income and assets, and that saving him from grave danger meant more in actual dollars to him than to a poor man. I finally gulped out: "I believe I should charge you $500." This seemed like a tremendous sum to me. Quick as a flash, Mr. X said: "I give you seven fifty!" And that was what he paid me. We became very good friends, and I later operated upon several members of his family. One day he gave me what he considered good business advice, namely, to get a better-looking car, as the one I had did not enhance my reputation. So I turned in my old Ford. At long last I had the courage to tell him about the "noiseless plate," and we had a good laugh over it.

Early in my private practice I considered it permissible before opening an abscess to inject a local anesthetic into the infected area. On one never-to-be-forgotten day, I had in the hospital a patient with an exquisitely painful abscess adjacent to the rectum, and I said to him: "Now, I am going to inject some Novocain so that you will feel no pain. You will feel just a little discomfort when the needle is introduced." I took the syringe which the nurse had prepared and injected a goodly quantity of fluid. Immediately, the patient began to yell loudly. What was my surprise, as I gazed at the abscess, to see it expand like an erupting volcano and blow off its top. By mistake I had been given a syringe full of hydrogen peroxide! Truly the abscess had been opened, dramatically, and the patient ultimately thanked me for the relief of his pain. However, I have never endorsed this method of opening an abscess.

Another time I was summoned to care for a workman in rough clothes whom I found bending over a fire hydrant. He was in evident agony and seemed unable to answer questions. I examined his abdomen as best I could under his shirt and found it to be rigid. Fearful that he had a perforated ulcer or some other serious condition, I put him in my car, rushed him to the hospital and did a laparotomy. Instead of finding a perforated ulcer as expected, I found nothing abnormal. I had been fooled by a malingerer.

I recall vividly the skillful manner in which Dr. Lewis Pollock exposed a certain malingerer. The man stoutly contended that he had unbearable pain and tenderness in the left flank and that he was unable to move his left leg. Pollock put on his stethoscope and listened to the man's heart, his face assuming such a serious expression of alertness and attention that the patient became fascinated in observing it. Meanwhile the patient was utterly unaware that Pollock was firmly and deeply palpating the allegedly tender flank. Cleverly, Pollock made no comment about this finding but inquired about the patient's left leg. "Sorry, Doc, I can't move it at all." "How is the right leg?" queried Pollock. "Fine!" said the patient and proved it by moving it briskly in all directions. Pollock asked if the right leg was strong enough to move upward if there was pressure on the knee? Pollock then placed both hands on the patient's right knee and put his full weight on it. The patient gave a mighty heave and raised the right leg, completely unaware of the fact that to effect this lift he had to brace himself by pressing strongly on the bed with the allegedly paralyzed leg. Pollock said nothing to the patient but wrote on the chart: "Feebleminded malingerer."

Another patient was a highly nervous, sensitive woman with severe suppurative tenosynovitis, gas anesthesia being required whenever the dressings were changed. As the original wound had been a puncture from a can opener, I thought it would be serving her best interests to give her some tetanus antitoxin. At that time, over thirty years ago, this involved the somewhat painful injection of 10 cc. of serum, which I carried out after changing the dressing and while the anesthetic was still in effect. The patient did not "come to" properly, and at first I thought the anesthetic had been improperly administered. Finally she became very cyanotic (blue) and almost pulseless, seeming about to die, when I heard her murmur the word "Adrenalin." This I promptly gave her, and she responded a little and finally recovered. It seems she was highly allergic to horse serum, and it was indeed a miracle that she had not died from the reaction to the tetanus antitoxin injection. Thereafter I always took great care to determine a patient's sensitivity before giving an injection.

One young woman, almost killed in an elevated train wreck on the north side of Chicago, was taken in profound shock to a nearby hospital, where I took care of her. She had numerous injuries, including a broken femur (thigh bone) and a head injury. A tremendous wound of her face and scalp had not been attended to because of her precarious general condition. Since a general anesthetic could not be given to her, I had to proceed with greatest gentleness and patience to shave her hair and cleanse the large wound of all street dirt. Then, as it is a less shocking procedure than taking stitches, I approximated the skin edges of the wound with many tiny bridges of adhesive tape. Fortunately, when the patient finally recovered, the scar on her face was quite inconspicuous.

One day two young girls were slowly riding in an automobile, one of them at the wheel, trying to decide what candies to select from a box, when their car suddenly crashed into a telephone pole. One girl sustained a dislocated hip, and for two days lay in a friend's house while a doctor of the "old school" frequently measured her legs, each time concluding with perplexity that they were

43

normal despite her intense pain. An x-ray easily settled the matter, and all ended happily after the dislocation was reduced at the hospital. Incidentally, the final blow for the girls was a bill from the Village of Winnetka for the broken telephone pole.

One night, about 2 A.M., I was summoned by a wealthy woman who was having a gallstone attack. I knew approximately the location of her huge residence, one of several mansions set far back from the main road and reached by a long, curving driveway. As I was driving along slowly, peering through the darkness for the proper driveway entrance, I was surprised to have a rough-looking man in shirt sleeves jump out from some bushes and try to flag me down. I did not stop for him, but drove on and turned into what I believed to be the right entrance, but soon I became increasingly doubtful of my whereabouts when I reached a wooden gate barring my passage. I got out, moved the gate aside, drove through and then dutifully closed the gate again, only to discover that I was at the edge of a cornfield. In order to turn the car around on the narrow road, I had to "back and fill" repeatedly. Before I knew it, the shirt-sleeved hitchhiker had opened the car door and had settled down beside me. While I was debating what my strategy should be, I was relieved to be able to analyze his voice and remarks and conclude that he was merely drunk. "Take me to the station," he muttered. Necessity accelerated my cerebration, and I quickly replied that he must first cooperate by getting out of the car and opening the wooden gate, which I had luckily closed. He docilely climbed out of the car and managed to hold the gate open while, like a flash, I sped past, leaving him standing there. After all, I had to hasten to my suffering patient!

The fact that superior intelligence in one field cannot always insure it in another, is borne out by the case of a certain appellate court judge. He called me at 3 o'clock one morning, almost exsanguinated from hemorrhage from the site of a hemorrhoid operation done the previous afternoon in a doctor's office!

In the case of a twelve-year-old girl who fell out of a tree and sustained a fracture of the spine, with complete paralysis of the lower extremities, I had to consult with a plumber. Together we contrived a longitudinal windlass over her bed with attachments to a special canvas-covered frame to support her. By means of this contraption the special nurse, who weighed less than the patient, could easily and unaided lift the patient in bed for nursing care.

I described this arrangement in an article published in *Surgery, Gynecology and Obstetrics* in April, 1925.

One especially difficult diagnosis was that of ruptured appendix in the schizophrenic son of a wealthy couple. This poor fellow had for years required tube feeding in a sanatorium. After I had operated on him and he had recovered from the dangerous appendiceal predicament, my pride was somewhat shaken by the remark of his psychiatrist: "You're a hell of a surgeon!"

One day sagacious Dr. "Andy" Aldrich called me to see a ten-year-old boy who was desperately ill with vomiting, some blood in the rectum and a large mass in the right side of the abdomen. The diagnosis was intussusception, which is a telescoping of part of the bowel into itself, an almost invariably fatal condition unless properly treated. Frequently an operation is necessary, but in some cases the bowel can be turned right side out by means of an enema (more recently a barium enema given under x-ray observation). After my arrival, Dr. Aldrich had another enema given, which happily resulted in a cure. Later, however, the parents were incensed to receive bills for house calls from two doctors for a child who "needed merely an enema."

A young lady who was making a short visit to Evanston was disturbed by the appearance of unsightly blue spots on her gums. So, she and her "boy friend" started at the top floor of the main doctors' office building hunting for someone who looked like a suitable doctor. By almost a miracle they chanced to visit the office of Dr. Wayne Fox, one of the best hematologists in this part of the country. He immediately recognized that she had an acute hemorrhagic purpura of the thrombocytopenic type, and at his insistence I did an emergency splenectomy that night. The operation was indeed a thriller, as bleeding was profuse until I could compress the splenic pedicle with thumb and forefinger and ligate it. The patient made a fine recovery.

At one time I took care of a boy of four years who had an ecchymotic mask, or traumatic asphyxia. The youngster had climbed into the family's car, which was parked on the gently sloping driveway to the house. Somehow he had released the brakes and then climbed out of the car and run behind it as it slowly rolled down the driveway. The boy's father happened to glance through a window and was horrified to see his little boy pinned to the ground, a rear wheel of the car crushing his chest. Miraculously, this frantic father summoned sufficient strength in his desperation to lift the 500 pound weight of the corner of the car, thus releasing his son and saving his life.

At the hospital one time while on rounds, I sent the nurse and interns out of the room as it was necessary to discuss some highly confidential matters with the patient. After about ten minutes, I was astonished to see a colored maid crawling out from under the bed. Apparently her curiosity had been sufficiently satisfied, and she wanted to leave.

Over the years I have taken care of many Christian Scientists, and for the most part they have been cooperative patients. There is much which is constructive and commendable in their philosophy, but it is regrettable that their fanaticism regarding medical problems plays such a prominent part. However, I have really admired some of the practitioners who have consulted me, and I feel that their vigor and cheerfulness have doubtless helped many a quaking personality. I recall one fine woman, in particular, who had broken bones in both legs and one arm. During her long stay at the hospital, while she was suspended in traction by ropes, pulleys and weights, we became well acquainted. One morning, as one professional addressing another, she asked: "How's *your* business, Doctor?" I replied that it was satisfactory. Whereupon she proudly volunteered the information that she had made $150 that week by telephoned "absent treatment" from her hospital bed. I venture to assume that she had not told her clients where she was located, but knowing her fine qualities, I believe that she gave them their full money's worth of help. Not long afterward, this practitioner wrote as follows:

> "I was so happy to read of your appointment as head of the surgery department at the hospital that I learned to love during my long visit there. My very splendid health today is largely due to what you knew and put into practice coupled with wonderful care. My sons and I are increasingly grateful to you. My heartiest congratulations for your success, well earned. . . ."

One of my most grateful patients was a Christian Scientist who had a huge ovarian cyst. It had become so large that its weight was a terrific burden to her emaciated body. After the simple operation for removal of the cyst, this woman regained her full health.

Well do I recall a certain woman who walked grimly into my office and demanded that I examine her ankle. Nothing seemed wrong with it. Thereupon she produced an x-ray picture of the ankle, and, again, nothing appeared to be wrong. I said, "The ankle is all right. Do not worry about it. Try to think of other, more pleasant subjects." Her face lit up with a bright smile as she said, "Well, that will be easy for me as I am a Christian Science practitioner!"

An excellent arrangement is possible if one parent is a Christian Scientist and the other is not. I recall one case in which the mother was a Scientist and the father was a Congregationalist. When their son broke a leg the mother told me that she had to humor her husband in the matter and summon a doctor. However, she refused to look at the x-rays of the fracture.

The worst *faux pas* I ever made was in the case of a woman weighing some two hundred and fifty pounds. She rushed breathlessly into the emergency room and imparted the dreadful information that she had sat on a needle. Indeed, a minute wound was visible in the appropriate area, and my heart sank, for I knew how difficult and sometimes futile a search for a needle can be. Soon, however, the x-ray picture gave the good news that the patient had been merely wounded and that no needle fragment remained. In my intense relief, I made the following naive statement: "Madam, you are very fortunate. The x-ray picture shows that your skin must have been merely pricked, as no fragment of needle is present. This is great luck, as otherwise it would have been like trying to find a needle in a haystack." From her cold look and the intern's efforts to suppress his mirth, I suddenly became aware that I had really chosen an unfortunate simile.

Certainly house calls bring the doctor into closer and more intimate association with patients and their families than the more formal office and hospital contacts, and I enjoyed countless pleasant and amusing incidents and anecdotes of a nonmedical nature. One time an elderly patient told me with pride about his grandson. It seems that the boy had appealed to his mother to wrap up a present he had purchased for his girl friend. "Why, Tommy," she said, "Do you mean to say that you paid fifty cents for this handkerchief?" Rather sheepishly the lad admitted that he had paid only twenty-five cents but had changed the price mark so as to make a more favorable impression on the recipient.

It is extremely useful to have a fund of stories with which to entertain and divert one's patients. Some stories may even have therapeutic value, but it is difficult to keep a fresh supply. The following are some of my old standbys: 1. Two small boys are talking. "My father is a doctor, and he keeps me well for nothing," says the first boy. The other retorts: "My father is a minister and he keeps me good for nothing." 2. A German band leader, trying to praise a band member who has repeatedly been tardy to rehearsals but had shown some improvement, says: "Mueller, you are early of late; you used to be behind before, but now you are first, at last." 3. The advice the doctor gave his patient in one of O'Henry's stories ("Let Me Feel Your Pulse"): "What you need is absolute rest and exercise."

One of my most harrowing experiences as a speaker occurred in the early days. Trying to be useful and public-spirited, I addressed a large group of girl scouts, who sat in open-mouthed respectful solemnity while I tried for an hour to make slings, splints and other first-aid subjects as thrilling as possible. When I stopped talking, there was a dead silence, which I finally unwisely broke by saying: "If any of you have any questions, I shall be glad to try to answer them." After some time, a little girl rose and shyly but with utmost seriousness inquired: "Could you tell me what makes my grandmother have gas on her stomach?" Evidently that was a serious problem in her household, and here was a chance for her to come home with glorious good tidings. For my part, I was non-plussed and soon dismissed the audience.

CHAPTER IV

The Patient Meets
the Surgeon

A PATIENT requiring an operation seldom comes to the surgeon directly, almost invariably being referred to the surgeon by a general practitioner or an internist. If the patient is ambulatory, he is referred to the surgeon's office, but if he has been admitted to the hospital, the surgeon will see him at the request of the internist for a surgical consultation. The referring physician must make up his mind that the case is definitely surgical or possibly surgical. In the latter event, many an internist may be prone to procrastinate. This is unfortunate, since he may evaluate too highly his own diagnostic and discriminatory powers and delay dangerously long in availing himself of the surgeon's experienced opinion. In a sense the internist's hesitation, while not uncommonly detrimental to the patient, is understandable. In some hospitals, unfortunately, surgical consultation usually means a pronouncement, which may be difficult to dispute, on the surgeon's part that an operation is mandatory, often immediately, rather than an exchange of views between internist and surgeon.

When a surgeon disagrees with an internist, he must speak up decisively, despite the fact that he may displease the internist by not accepting his diagnosis. Naturally the surgeon must lean heavily on the internist in the appraisal of the surgical risk, based on the capacity of the heart and blood vessels, the kidneys and the liver to withstand the operation.

After an operation the internist usually leaves the principal care of the patient to the surgeon, and sees the patient only in a friendly and encouraging capacity, not writing any orders unless invited to do so by the surgeon. Only one person can have full responsibility and authority after an operation, and that must be the surgeon. His task is indeed trying during the postoperative course if the internist takes an active, independent part in the patient's care, even to the extent of changing the surgeon's orders. However, patience and forebearance will usually see one through. Needless to say, an internist often makes valuable suggestions, which should be gratefully accepted. In most instances, a surgeon sees a patient during only one episode, while an internist may see him many times over a period of years and the term "my patient" acquires such increasing possessiveness that the patient himself may become uncomfortably aware of the situation.

A general practitioner, or "generalist," often has some justifiable complaints about surgeons in general and about some surgeons in particular. The hidden drama of the operating room often overemphasizes the part which the surgeon plays in a patient's recovery. The surgeon's stature is magnified in the patient's eyes, and his fee, though large, may be cheerfully paid, while grumbling arises over the internist's fee (usually smaller), although the internist actually may have saved the patient's life by making the correct diagnosis and promptly insuring the receipt of the proper surgical treatment.

Frequently a surgeon must withdraw from a hopeless case of cancer after an operation has achieved "everything possible" to save the patient's life, and with relief he turns the patient over to the referring physician. Occasionally, a certain type of surgeon may make the medical man's task far more difficult by "successfully" performing some extensive, mutilating operation which has but slight chance of prolonging the patient's existence. Often the surgeon crosses the scene of some illness briefly; it is the general practitioner or the internist who must plod along to the end of a task that draws increasingly upon his patience, his strength and his ability to encourage the patient and his family.

The patient himself, or certainly his medical counselor, should know something of the approximate percentage of probability of life prolongation with and without operation in various stages of a disease. Such statistics are difficult to obtain, and not many surgeons know them, but they should supply them on demand. For instance: What are the percentage chances of longevity in cancer of the lung which has spread to the adjacent lymph nodes, with and without operation? What is the relative suffering of the patient? What is the cost? No positive answers can be given, but the probabilities must be thoroughly discussed and carefully considered.

Often the diagnosis offers little problem, as in the case of hernia, breast tumor or cancer of the rectum. When the internist has made the diagnosis at his office, he informs the patient that an operation will be necessary and asks him if he has a preference as to a surgeon. Sometimes the patient will name a surgeon whom the internist deems competent, and the referral is decided at once. More often the patient will ask the internist whom he would recommend. The internist usually names two or three men whom he believes suitable, naturally naming his first choice first. How the internist determines upon his first choice may involve a complicated pattern of thought and experience. Actually he is not ideally equipped to evaluate the quality of a surgeon's work. He has had virtually no surgical experience, and rarely takes the time to watch an operation from beginning to end, perhaps spending only a few minutes in the operating room. For an evaluation of a surgeon's skill, judgment and temperament, the collected opinions of his five most recent residents would be most accurate.

Naturally, an internist is strongly influenced in his appraisal of a surgeon by the opinions expressed by a patient after an operation is finished. He does not want to be reproached for having chosen a surgeon whom the patient does not like. The internist, properly, is chiefly influenced by the surgeon's record of successful experience in each particular type of operation, but he is usually not able to make fine distinctions, one surgeon being as good as another in the internist's eyes. Moreover, the internist is not immune to "the line" displayed by some surgeons. A solemn, authoritative manner in a situation not intimately familiar to the internist frequently carries more than its justifiable weight. Many surgeons learn to exhibit a hearty, assured manner, which the internists assume is a reflection of the proper temperament for a surgeon.

The best method for insurance of referral of patients by an internist is for the surgeon to give skillful, courteous and gentle treatment to every patient, to inform the referring internist completely about all the details of any operation, and to evidence his actual experience by means of presentations before medical meetings or by publications. After every operation the surgeon should write a personal letter to the referring internist and enclose a detailed account of the operation, a carbon copy of the report of the pathologic specimen and any other pertinent details which will help the internist in the future care of the patient.

The patient's first meeting with the surgeon is of great importance. Often, in the first few minutes, the patient makes up his mind about the character and abilities of his surgeon-to-be. All types of patients visit the doctor, and his manner of winning their confidence varies with their education, temperament and state of apprehension. Friendliness, patience and attentive interest in the patient's story are essential. But one must not forget the merit in Burrows'[24] slightly cynical remark: "The public are so lacking in discernment that it matters not how much or how little a man may know provided he has the qualities of plausibility and persuasiveness." Moreover, one cannot, for practical reasons, agree with Plato's pronouncement, which was echoed by Montaigne, that "good doctors themselves ought to have had the diseases they want to cure."

Many times in my first conversation with a patient I have said: "What is your difficulty?" To which the patient has replied: "That's for you to find out, Doc." Such an answer is due partly to what he considers witty self-assurance and what he fancies to be shrewdness that will not mislead the doctor to any preformed opinion. One doctor is purported to have replied to such a retort: "If you will excuse me just a minute, I will be back with a veterinarian. He's the only one I know who can make a diagnosis without asking questions."

Admittedly, the patient must tell the story of why he came to the doctor and when he first noticed that something was wrong—pain, abnormal function, a lump, a bloody discharge. The manner in which the patient presents his complaint reveals much concerning his emotional make-up. On one side is the patient whose complaints are obviously largely imaginary, while on the other side is the patient typified by the man who had suffered from pain and vomiting all night because he "didn't want to disturb" the surgeon. John Homans[29] has made these comments on what constitutes a "good" or a "bad" patient:

"A good patient is one who has an interesting ailment capable of cure and at the same time continues to look pleasant, understands directions, asks very few questions and never complains. A bad patient begins by telling a poor story, full, not of fact, but of the alleged opinions of many physicians, is not easy of diagnosis and contrives to irritate and bewilder the attendants. Such a patient complains continually, asks questions innumerable, and whether things go well or ill, never gives the attendants the satisfaction of seeing her made happy. There are, of course, degrees of badness. Some patients are terrible, while others are just difficult. The truth is that they are all sick."

In some instances, as in a case of hernia, the entire matter of the operation can be settled at one visit. In others, such as cases of suspected gallstones or of intestinal tumor, various x-rays and laboratory tests will have to be made before a final decision can be reached as to the need and wisdom of operating. It is my preference to examine for hernia first with the patient standing while I am seated. I am always gentle and considerate and, for my own protection, ask the patient to turn his head sideways before coughing to help demonstrate the presence of a hernia. Then I usually examine the patient while he lies down. Parenthetically, I might say, it practically never fails that if a patient is asked to lie down on the table, he will lie on his back, but if he is told to lie on his back, he will, for some unknown reason, lie on his stomach. It is extremely important to have a nurse present during the examination of a female patient, both out of consideration for the patient and for protection of the doctor. Also, it is highly desirable to avoid making a quick diagnosis, as one will naturally tend to try to fit symptoms into a preconceived pattern. The best method is to defer making a diagnosis until all the necessary tests and examinations have been completed.

After a diagnosis has been made, it is the doctor's duty to explain the situation in simple terms, patiently telling why surgical treatment is indicated, the type of operation required, the average length of time the patient will need to be away from work and the probability of cure. Next the questions of hospital accommodations, special nurses and the surgeon's fee (referred to later) are discussed. At this point the patient may say that, while he has confidence in your doing the operation, he feels that he should have a confirmatory opinion from another surgeon, and such a request should always be met. The only reservation that I insist upon is that the consultant be a man at least as experienced as I am in the particular problem involved, and preferably of greater experience. I usually give the patient the names of three or four surgeons whose ability I respect. If he questions the impartiality of my recommendations, I suggest that he call the dean of the medical school or the administrator of a large hospital for the name of a consultant. If the consultant disagrees with the original diagnosis, a third consultant may have to be called, or the unfortunate patient may make the decision on the basis of his own knowledge of the medical problem.

As suggested previously, one's remarks to a patient necessarily vary with his intelligence and with the type of operation required. For example, the following is a paraphrase of what I usually say to a man with an inguinal hernia:

> "You have an inguinal hernia, commonly called a rupture, on the right side. I have examined the left side but find none there. This type of hernia is an enlargement of the ring in the abdominal wall through which the spermatic cord passes. This enlargement makes a weak place in the wall, allowing the abdominal contents to protrude through in varying degree according to the size of the weakened area.
>
> "A man in your situation has four alternatives to consider. The first is to do nothing about the hernia. However, this alternative is excluded since the hernia if untreated will become larger, will cause more discomfort, will interfere with your capacity for physical exercise and sports, will not disappear spontaneously and may even become caught and result in strangulation of the loop of intestine. While strangulated hernia is a relatively uncommon complication, every large hospital has a number of cases each year. Unless the patient is given the relief afforded by an emergency operation, the outcome is fatal."

I usually minimize the likelihood of strangulation, as the risk is small, especially in urban communities where the patient can be given prompt help. Moreover, it is best to try to give the facts as accurately as possible and certainly not give the patient the impression that he is being scared into having an operation.

I then continue the preliminary discussion:

> "The second alternative is the injection treatment. I mention this only to condemn it, and because some of your friends may have advised you that it is an easy way to avoid an operation. Some twenty years ago the medical schools of the University of Minnesota, Northwestern University and other universities thoroughly investigated this

method and repudiated it. I believe the injection treatment is more difficult to carry out than an operation. But the outstanding argument against this method is that in a carefully studied large series of cases at a distinguished New York hospital, the rate of recurrence was at least 84 per cent.

"The third and fourth alternatives are to wear a truss or to have an operation, and the patient *must* do one or the other. I recommend an operation. In many instances a man has worn a truss for twenty or thirty years and has become as used to it as to his shoes, but in most cases the man who insists that he will not have an operation and will use a truss actually discards it in about a week. The disadvantages of a truss are numerous. First, it will not cure the hernia. In infants a hernia may often be cured by a truss, but the efforts to keep the truss in place are harrowing, and operation has usually supplanted this method. The second disadvantage of the truss is that it protects only when properly fitted and properly worn and, moreover, only while it is being worn. Practically every man removes the truss at night and is therefore unprotected when he jumps out of bed to close a window or to get up in the morning. The third disadvantage is that a truss is almost always uncomfortable, and its pressure on the skin often produces painful irritation or inflammation. Finally, many men object to having their infirmity advertised when dressing in a golf club locker room or gymnasium.

"The fourth alternative, and the one I usually recommend, is operation. Admittedly, a hernia operation does not offer a 100 per cent assurance of cure. Several years ago I made a careful follow-up study of a large group of my cases which I had reported in the surgical literature. In all of these cases the same type of operation was used, regardless of the size of the hernia or the patient's age, and the incidence of recurrence proved to be 3.1 per cent. Therefore, a patient who agrees to have a hernia operation has at least a 96 per cent prospect of a cure. Even in the rare event of recurrence, a second operation can be done but offers a somewhat lower percentage prospect of cure than for the first operation.

"Naturally, you are concerned about the risk of an operation, since no operation is entirely devoid of it, but in hernia operations the risk is extremely slight. Likewise no ride on a train or in an automobile is devoid of risk, but no one is deterred from riding because of this. In the case of a hernia, the risk of doing nothing is greater than the risk of the operation, to say nothing of the discomfort and limitation of activities that are relieved by operation.

"I shall expect you to be able to stand beside the bed on the day of the operation and certainly to walk a little the next day. A general anesthetic will be used, and as soon as you wake up you should make a point of moving your feet many times, since it is of great importance to insure proper circulation following operation. You will feel pain in the wound, especially upon movement, but the wound is strong. You should move about freely and must cough up any mucus in the throat, even if it does increase the pain temporarily. You may expect to leave the hospital on the third to the sixth day and to be away from office work for about two weeks. You may drive your car in from seven to ten days after the operation if difficult parking and sudden stops are avoided. Golf may be started in three weeks and tennis six weeks after the operation. If possible, you should always avoid heavy lifting (100 pounds or more)."

Often the patient will ask: "As a matter of interest, Doctor, just exactly how do you do this operation? Tell me in plain, common sense English!" This poses a dilemma. The patient's knowledge of anatomy and the terms descriptive of the surgical procedures will render an account as intelligible to him as the explanation of analytical geometry to a grade school child. Usually the patient is satisfied by the statement that "the weak area is sewed over in layers and made strong," but if he insists on having all details, I tell him, with entire truth, that I did not understand the anatomical details of a hernia and its repair until after I had graduated from medical school and was "scrubbed up" at the operating table.

In performing a herniotomy, too much care cannot be taken to insure against the error of operating upon the wrong side. (See the chapter on Surgical Pitfalls.)

One of the most trying duties of a surgeon is that of telling a patient he will be required to have a permanent colostomy after an operation, for instance, in a case of cancer of the rectum. The devastating fact must be presented in as kindly, sympathetic and optimistic a manner as possible. Nurses are the worst counselors in this regard, as they have had the disagreeable task of caring for a colostomy in its early stages, before its relatively clean management is established. I recall one fine nurse who, in her ignorance, elected death from the disease rather than have a permanent colostomy. Often I am able to state definitely that a colostomy will not need to be permanent. In a few cases I must reserve final judgment until the operation is being performed, so the patient will simply have to depend upon my judgment at that time.

When convinced that a colostomy is unavoidable I say something like this:

> "In order to eradicate this growth, it will be necessary to remove the rectum entirely, and you will always have to have bowel movements through an opening in the abdominal wall (colostomy). Your natural reaction of distaste to this unpleasant information is all out of proportion to the actual facts. When you learn that in most cases a

person with a colostomy can continue all of his business and social activities without anyone's knowing about his condition, and when you know that the care of a colostomy is minimal, you will feel much more relieved at your prospects."

A person with a colostomy has a bowel movement by means of an enema every day or once in two or three days, depending on his preference. He takes an enema while seated on the toilet, using a specially designed apparatus. No assistance is necessary, and he usually prefers to be entirely independent. An enema may be taken in the morning or in the evening, depending on convenience, and between times no bag or apparatus is worn over the colostomy. The patient follows a relatively constipating diet, according to a detailed list that is given to him, and after several months the new opening will function smoothly and without annoyance. I always tell a patient, in anticipation of contrary advice from friends, that the care of this abdominal type of colostomy is relatively simple, while that of a perineal colostomy is usually a nightmare. Despite the claims of the proponents of a perineal colostomy that some muscular (sphincter) control is possible, such control is almost always a failure, and daily cleanliness and digital dilatation cannot be obtained as well as with an abdominal wall colostomy. I always provide the patient with a set of mimeographed instructions, including the detailed diet list, which will enable him to control the bowel movements.

For years I have been waiting for a patient to ask me, "Just how many times have you done this operation, Doctor?" but the question has still to be asked. However, I am ready for it, as I have kept an analytic record of my surgical experience in over 5,000 major operations.

I am often asked to do highly specialized operations in which I have had no experience, such as neurologic surgery, thoracic surgery, and surgery for cleft palate and harelip. Invariably patients requiring these operations are referred to men who are skilled in these specialties (see the discussion of Specialization).

CHAPTER V

Nonoperative Hospital Activities

I N CONSIDERING the surgeon's activities at the hospital, those out- side of the operating room will be dealt with first. It is impor- tant for the surgeon to register in and out of the hospital promptly without fail, so that important messages can reach him. In some hospitals the incoming surgeon moves a switch opposite his name on an electric board. This lights up his name on several boards throughout the hospital, including the one in the main telephone office from which paging calls originate. If he fails to sign out when leaving the hospital, he greatly complicates the telephone operator's work. It has seemed to me that certain doctors "forget" oftener than others; as a result they are paged endlessly, thus giving an exaggerated impression of professional activity. This maneuver is much like that of a young practitioner in a small town years ago who used to drive his horse and buggy furiously through the main street every once in a while, even though going nowhere in par- ticular. It is desirable for the surgeon to arrive at the hospital as nearly as possible at the same time each day and follow the same route through the hospital. This will enable interns and residents to meet him more quickly. Often, of course, more attending men are visiting their patients in the hospital at the same time than there are interns to accompany them. The house staff endeavor to meet with as many attending men as possible, both to learn from them and to be of service to them.

The visiting of patients by a doctor is dignified by the term "rounds" if there are enough patients. Rounds usually start at the head nurse's office, where the patients' charts are kept. Careful scrutiny, contemplation and discussion of the charts is one of the physician's heaviest responsibilities and intellectual exercises. The many detailed entries since his last visit must be studied, clarified if necessary, and evaluated. Often it is necessary to review the entire chart in order to appraise the significance of new data. Temperature, pulse, respiration, blood pressure, output of urine, defecation, passage of gas, dyspnea, coughing, degree of activity, and intake of fluids by mouth, vein or proctoclysis must be considered. Laboratory reports must be studied to determine a patient's electrolyte needs; figures for gas and fluids when continuous gastric suction is employed must be analyzed, and blood counts and blood chemistry determinations must be heeded. The medications which have been given and their effects, if recognizable, must be noted.

A campaign for treatment of each patient for the next twenty-four hours must be decided upon and the orders clarified with interns and nurses. This latter duty is usually attended to after the patient has been visited. These activities require the closest application and deep thought, corresponding, I should think, to the high level conferences in a law firm in deciding the strategy in momentous pieces of litigation, or the meetings of the executive committee of a large corporation to decide upon an important change of business policy. As a rule, the conferences of lawyers and business men are held in the undisturbed quiet of a high executive's office, protected from intrusions of people and telephone calls. Considered opinions can be voiced without interruption.

The decisions a doctor must make at the head nurse's office often require the same degree of concentration and cogitation as those of the lawyers and business men, but in what a different environment must he make them! The loud speaker is incessantly paging physicians; the telephone rings over and over again before a nurse can answer some perhaps trivial question; student nurses, proud of their new responsibility in charting minor information, snatch charts from every direction, trying at times to make entries in the charts that the doctor is trying to study. Worst of all are the breezy and facetious interruptions of colleagues who stroll in and whose patients are not sufficiently ill to require serious concentration. "Well, how's the old golf game, Bill?" often shatters a train of thought. I must admit that the confusion in the head nurse's office has always been too much for me, and unless it is merely to inspect the course in a case in which convalescence is smooth, I prefer to take the chart and with the resident and intern try to find a quiet, peaceful corner in the hospital where we can give vital matters our deliberate, undivided attention.

The primary purposes of visiting a patient in the hospital are, first, to appraise his physical condition and search out the possibilities for helping him; and, second, to convey to him encouragement and spiritual uplift. It is a matter of considerable judgment to determine the degree by which these objectives are aided or hindered by the number of the house staff who accompany the surgeon on his rounds and what conversation can be had with them in the patient's presence. At times it may be best for the surgeon to visit a patient alone. After a patient has become somewhat accustomed to the house staff, particularly after the intern has taken his history, it is usually profitable for the house staff to listen to your conversation with a patient and observe how you dress his wound. Certainly all profound discussion of the pros and cons of the diagnosis and treatment, while educational to the house staff, must be conducted outside the patient's room and not within earshot. Patients differ in their reactions to having the surgeon accompanied by two or more "men in white suits." Some, especially when convalescent, find it entertaining and complimentary that their cases are of interest. Others resent the presence of a retinue as an invasion of their privacy. Tact and judgment on the doctor's part are required to combine the maximum help for the patient and the maximum instruction for the house staff. Occasionally, in an especially interesting case a patient may be presented before a roomful of medical students, but only if his full consent has been obtained.

Many an intern, unfortunately, comes to regard the hospital patient very impersonally as an exhibit put there solely for educational purposes. He is prone to become lost in the professional aspects of the case. Such an attitude results in disadvantage not only to the patient but also to the intern, for he may tend to acquire an unsympathetic manner of questioning and examination which will diminish his value to patients and will be a deterrent to him in the development of his private practice. This is one of the pitfalls of an internship in a large urban charity hospital.

Much may be said for the "teaching hospital." Such a hospital is affiliated with a medical school, is staffed by members of the medical school faculty and stresses the instruction and training of medical students and house staff. But it is not an unmixed blessing. I am inclined to think that the most vocal of the proponents of the teaching hospitals are the leaders in the medical schools who eloquently extol the advantages of medical school affiliation in assuring patients of the most up-to-date and alert care. The constant association with the medical school faculty and the intellectual stimulation furnished by the "profound" and searching questions of the third and fourth year medical students and house staff are claimed to keep the physician "on his toes." True, the patient often does benefit, but the physician may be especially stimulated by the necessity of convincing his medical colleagues and superiors that he is keeping up. Alas, much of his time may have to be spent preparing for and giving lectures on subjects about which he is not presently concerned. Relieved of this time-taking obligation, if he is properly constituted, he would have more time to study his individual patients and engage in clinical research.

Some leaders in medical schools are naturally pleased when they can expound with regard to hospital affiliations and teaching plans. By their reports to associations of deans and medical teachers and university boards of trustees, their own stature is increased, while irreproachably proclaiming the great good to the sick of their teaching methods. These are the men who have the ear of hospital boards and university boards. While their leadership generally is wise, it is certainly not infallible, and their motives are not entirely disinterested. Basically, the prime function of the physician is care of the sick; if this be so, the leaders argue, the education of the physician transcends all other responsibilities. There is danger in carrying this line of reasoning too far, for one might go so far as to say that the physician's automobile or other means of transportation is the most important factor, for without it he would not be able to see his patients. Understandably, Wartman[30] refers to "the fear that the expert in (medical) education, although always enthusiastic as to methods, may sometimes be sterile as to knowledge."

Competition in medicine, by and large, makes for better medical care, just as competition in auto manufacture and airplane building makes for better products. The hard core of medical competition is the care of the sick. He who cures or relieves the most patients in the most expeditious and sympathetic manner should and almost always is the most successful in his practice. But, in this connection, it is well to reflect upon the remarks of Walton Hale Hamilton,[28] who said:

> "The incidence of competitive medical enterprise falls heavily upon all the parties concerned. Although 'the personal choice of a physician' is an excellent ideal, it does not, under current conditions, work well in practice. An old maxim, long known to every student of social philosophy, calls for a restriction of personal choice when 'the consumer is not a proper judge of the quality of the ware.' The art of medicine is intricate; the relation of the treatment of the sick to results obtained cannot be appraised by the layman; in medicine, almost more certainly than anywhere else, the patient has not the knowledge requisite for judgment. In almost every city reputable physicians will admit—at least in private—that the competence of their fellows is not in accord with their respective reputations."

With the complicating factor of the medical school faculty and the teaching hospital staff membership, the physician's energies and fortunes become inextricably involved in competition of a different nature. He must impress his medical school and hospital colleagues by making contributions to medical knowledge. A few men make solid additions and many who try to do so actually improve their minds by the study and effort involved; but still others are wasting their time. Councils of medical schools passing upon promotions and leaders on hospital staffs are increasingly falling into the questionable habit of judging candidates on the mere number of their publications. Certainly this practice is the greatest incentive to the production of mediocre work. If, as occasionally happens, the judges themselves have attained their positions of eminence by the quantity rather than the quality of their own efforts, the vicious circle is enlarged. Moreover, the hard-working man whose chief objective is the care of the sick and whose waking hours are chiefly spent in studying to increase his ability to care for the sick will come to be patronized and looked down upon by the so-called "leaders." It must never be lost sight of that the good clinician is the cornerstone of sound medical care. If the physician, in addition to being a good clinician, can make a judicious contribution to the literature, his usefulness will be increased. Admittedly, the optimum functioning of this man is augmented by the widely diversified work of all the research scientists. It is to be hoped, therefore, that hospital staffs have an equable balance of clinical and research teachers, or, best, that the finest qualities of each type are included in each individual.

The hospital staff is required to have a constitution and by-laws which have been approved by the lay board. A great part of the staff work can be delegated to committees whose authority has staff backing.

To insure the highest possible standard of professional work, the staff should adopt some type of annual staff audit. The American College of Surgeons[31] is studying plans for such appraisals. To my mind such an audit would be compiled from a formula which includes properly weighed consideration of the number of hospital patients, the hospital mortality, the percentage of necropsy permits, the length of hospital stay (according to illness or injury?), the number of consultations, the discrimination shown in ordering laboratory work, the attention to completion of hospital records, the ability to insure good intern service, the amount of time spent in teaching nurses' classes, the significant contributions to medical literature, time spent in free clinics, service on staff committees and cooperation with social service workers.

Myers and Slee[32] define a "medical audit" as

". . . the evaluation by physicians of the quality of patient care, as revealed by the medical records, in order that four questions may be answered. (1) What did the patient have? (2) What was done for him? (3) Was the treatment optimum? (4) If not, why not? The answers obtained, when collected, tabulated and analyzed, provide a means of evaluating the care of a single patient or of groups of patients and afford a method of documenting the performance of doctors, individually and collectively. . . . Any method which does not include the judgment of physicians is not a medical audit."

Myers and Slee conclude, in part, that "the medical staff of any hospital is qualified to conduct its own medical audit. . . . One category of disease or operation should be evaluated during a single audit period."

Lembcke[33] has contributed an important article entitled "Medical Auditing by Scientific Methods." In his summary he states:

"To place medical auditing on a scientific basis it is necessary to (1) employ uniform definitions for classifying diagnosis and treatment;

(2) verify statements in the clinical record by means of written reports of laboratory examination or of consultation, or by other forms of documentation; (3) determine whether the pathology, x-ray, and other clinical laboratory reports on which many of the criteria are based are comparable in accuracy and terminology with those of control hospitals; (4) judge results according to objective criteria; and (5) measure the degree of compliance with criteria against standards derived from observations in control hospitals."

He describes in detail the application of these methods to major female pelvic surgery and finds that:

". . . they can be highly effective in bringing to light and helping to correct situations where the type of operation is unsuitable or the diagnostic study is inadequate and especially where the number of operations is excessive."

A recent development in the matter of review is the newly recognized "Tissue Committee" fostered by the American College of Surgeons and adopted by the Joint Commission on Accreditation of Hospitals. Myers[34] defines this committee as "a committee of the medical staff of a hospital, which evaluates the surgery done by the medical staff and rates the competence of each surgeon on the basis of his performance." He adds,

"For the proper functioning of the tissue committee, several essentials must be present: 1. A co-operative medical staff which desires to have the surgical work audited and is willing to perform this often unpleasant task. 2. A tissue committee composed of appointed members of the medical staff who are responsible to the executive committee and the medical staff. 3. A pathologist who is competent, honest and forthright. He should preferably not be the chairman of the tissue committee. 4. The requirement that all surgical tissue shall be sent to the pathologist for examination. 5. An executive committee and medical staff willing to discipline those surgeons whose work is found to deviate consistently from accepted standards."

Elsewhere Myers[35] says:

"The sole function of the tissue committee of the medical staff is to establish the justification for surgery done at the hospital. It can accomplish this purpose by one means only: The evaluation by physicians of all clinical indications for surgery in each individual case. There is at present no other valid method for making this decision. The pathologist's tissue diagnosis alone is not the yardstick of the justification for surgery, and a normal tissue rate (the ratio of normal tissue removed to the total number of surgical procedures done) is likewise invalid for this purpose." (See also the chapter on Surgical Pitfalls.)

In 1949, my senior resident in surgery, Dr. Theodore T. Myre, examined between 15,000 and 20,000 cards in the Evanston Hospital record room in order to make a survey of the work done by the members of the Department of Surgery. A study of the surgical mortality at the hospital for the 136-month period from July 1, 1929, to November 1, 1940, was compared with the 105-month period from November 1, 1940, to August 1, 1949. Only the commoner, standard operations were used as a basis for comparison, but all of these operations for those periods were included regardless of the patient's age, the risk involved or the severity of the surgical condition. If death occurred from any cause, regardless of the length of time following an operation, it was considered to be a "surgical death" if the patient had not left the hospital.

The compiled statistics were summarized in the hospital magazine, *The Pilot,* in the May, 1950, number, as follows:

> "In the years since 1940, safety for a patient undergoing any one of six standard operations at Evanston Hospital has been four times greater than it was in the previous ten years. The six operations covered by these figures are: 1. appendectomy; 2. cholecystectomy, or gallbladder operation; 3. herniorrhaphy, or hernia operation; 4. thyroidectomy, or removal of the thyroid gland; 5. radical breast amputation, and, 6. Rammstedt operation, or the opening of an obstruction (present at birth) from the stomach to the intestines in young infants. The mortality rate for the 4,720 operations performed since November 1, 1940, has been on an average of 6.1 deaths per 1,000 as compared with the average of previous years of 24.8 per 1,000."

From July 3, 1946, to January 1, 1950, there were 1,186 consecutive appendectomies without a death, and from February 1, 1946, to January 1, 1950, there were 310 consecutive cholecystectomies without a death. Moreover, in this study a careful record was made of the number and mortality of each of the standard operations done by all the surgeons doing the principal amount of work. In this way it was ascertained how many of each of the operations the various surgeons were performing and what their over-all mortality was for the two periods under comparison. I had mimeographed copies of these studies prepared and distributed to all the members of the surgical department.

One of the surgeon's most important responsibilities is to talk with the anxious waiting relatives after an operation. If the start of the operation is delayed or if the operation itself is unduly prolonged, I try to send a message to the family that all is well, since there is probably no more trying ordeal than waiting for several hours while a relative is in the operating room. No matter how tired the surgeon is, no matter how far behind he is in his schedule and no matter how long since he has had anything to eat, he must patiently and in some detail recount the details of the operation to the family. First of all, they must be assured that the patient withstood the operation satisfactorily. I usually start by saying:

> "He went through the operation very well and his present condition is very satisfactory. He is now in the recovery room, where specially trained attendants will care for him until he is returned to his hospital bed. We have succeeded in doing what was necessary, and we are very optimistic that the patient will rapidly regain his full health."

It may be necessary to report to the family that something different was found than was anticipated, or even that, despite the definite indications for operation, no condition requiring surgical treatment was found. For instance, I have had to tell a family that the patient's appendix was normal and that the cause of the trouble was inflammation of the lymph nodes of the intestinal mesentery—a condition which often cannot be differentiated from acute appendicitis preoperatively. I have had to report failure to find a suspected displaced semilunar cartilage of the knee. Unfortunately it is frequently necessary to report that an inoperable malignant growth was found or that only a palliative operation could be done.

No matter what the operation has been, two of the commonest questions asked by the family are: "Was everything else all right? Was there any sign of cancer?" To the first question, I believe the correct answer to be: "In the area in which I was operating I saw nothing abnormal, and I did not consider it wise to risk unwanted complications by searching about in the abdomen when there were no indications for doing so." In the second instance, when there is no actual sign of cancer, it is important to state this fact so definitely as to leave no doubt in anyone's mind.

What to tell the patient with cancer is a difficult question, no simple answer being possible. Each surgeon will have to decide for himself what is best in each case since, even among men of the highest professional and ethical standards, no agreement has been reached. I have seen a group of some ten leading surgeons and physicians at an informal meeting discussing this problem and their opinions were about equally divided as to the proper solution. On one side was a distinguished surgeon who intoned loudly, and with evident parade of virtue: "There is no substitute for the truth!" On the other side of the argument, a wise old physician told of the case of a physician friend who was found to have a malignant tumor of the eye, which proved fatal in a year. The patient was told that the condition was innocent, and he continued his professional work almost to the end. Those who knew his temperament felt that, had he known the truth, his last year of life would have been spent in melancholy idleness, insupportable to himself and to his family, rather than hopefully in his accustomed useful occupation.

The late L. J. Henderson, a noted Harvard biological chemist, once said: "The notion that the truth, the whole truth, and nothing but the truth can be conveyed to the patient is a good specimen of that class of fallacies called by Whitehead 'the fallacy of misplaced concreteness.' " Many factors must be considered. When questionnaires are sent out to large groups of well people asking them what they would want to be told, almost invariably the reply is a courageous and resounding "the truth!" But "when the chips are down," the doomed person usually prefers otherwise. The age of the patient, his family responsibilities, his emotional make-up and the family relationships must be considered. No two patients and no two families are alike and the doctor must try to develop Solomon-like sagacity.

Most families importune the doctor not to tell the patient when cancer is discovered. Louis J. Regan,[36] one-time professor of legal medicine in California, once said:

> "It is extremely doubtful if a physician has a therapeutic privilege to withhold a specific diagnosis from a patient with serious or fatal illness. On the contrary, it appears to be clear that, in ordinary circumstances, the confidential relation requires that the physician make a frank and full disclosure when his patient is adult and mentally competent."

Most of the published statements of surgeons and physicians on this subject affirm that the patient should be told that he has a fatal disease even though a considerable, indefinite interval may intervene before his death. By making such a statement, certainly the doctor clears himself of any possible legal risk, and he can boast that his conscience is clear because he tells the truth! But, alas, this conventionally correct act, while enabling the surgeon to shrug his shoulders, may crush the patient and his family under an almost insupportable burden. In many cases I have cared for a patient who has been fatally ill with cancer but who has been mercifully spared that knowledge and, until he lapsed into final unconsciousness, was made to feel that he was getting better. I have always been proud when I have succeeded in making a patient feel this way or at least have encouraged his optimistic outlook. In one of the few instances in which I had about decided to tell a man that he had widespread cancer of the liver, his wife, at a private conference with me, said reproachfully: "You would be giving him the death sentence!" I therefore changed my tactics, and for months this patient was cheerful and optimistic, attributing his lack of well-being to an unusually slow convalescence from the operation. Finney[2] says: "The true province of the doctor has been well stated by the late Dr. E. L. Trudeau: 'To cure sometimes, to relieve often, to comfort always!'"

I feel that Warren Cole[37] has stated the problem most admirably in the following words:

> "I wish to bring up another controversial point about lay education, namely, the question as to whether patients should be told when they have a cancer. I do not believe this question can be answered categorically. Each patient should be individualized. Some people are so apprehensive that this knowledge would make the rest of their life miserable. Under such circumstances I believe it is better to be completely frank only with some responsible member of the family; the patient can be told he has a growth which must be removed lest it invade the body. However, on many occasions, business men will ask you to be sure to tell them if they have a cancer which might result in their premature death. Under such circumstances, and assuming we are dealing with a fairly stable individual, I am convinced we should be frank for two reasons: In the first place it is usually very important in the future care of the patient's family for the head of the family to be aware of the possibility of a premature death; in the second place such people usually have enough strength of character to adjust to this knowledge, and live the rest of their lives without jeopardizing their emotional stability. When metastases develop and the patient is aware of their possible significance, I strongly emphasize that after we have utilized and perhaps exhausted our therapeutic measures we make strong psychologic use of the fact that occasionally malignant

tumors spontaneously stop growing. Under such circumstances most people are surprisingly content so long as they know there is a possibility the tumor will be brought under control, even though that possibility is remote. The medical profession has not made proper use of this valuable asset in allaying the fears and apprehension of the patient or relatives."

After examining the ethics of this question, I have concluded that the best guide is to adopt such a course as will give the patient (not the doctor) the maximum of happiness. Generally speaking, I have not told a patient he has cancer, even in response to a direct question, or at least have grossly understated the peril. Unless he has heavy financial responsibilities, or important legal matters to settle, such as revising a will or making changes in his business organization, I do not believe it helps either him or his family to tell him that he is doomed to certain death. If he can still have a ray of hope, even if it is faint and remote, he is much strengthened in his resolve to show courage, patience and kindliness. Moreover, a patient may actually know the truth but may choose to pretend to be deceived. This gallant role makes it far easier for his visits with his family, which is perhaps the most important facet of the problem. The husband and wife, or other relatives, see and talk to each other many times daily. Sad indeed if their conversation must deal with or be haunted by the certainty of death. How much happier for them if the surgeon says: "Well, this has been a bad day, but tomorrow will be better," or, "We'll get this thing licked!" Moreover, who knows, the scientific world may be startled on some tomorrow by the news that a chemical cure for cancer has been found.

In many instances I have told a patient, for example when cancer of the breast or of the colon has been discovered, that a "few cancer cells" were found, but the entire area was widely removed. I tell each patient that he is fortunate that the disease was discovered early and that he is *cured*. Indeed, in many cases a cure does follow operation. Usually such a patient will ask, "Is there any possibility that this will ever come back?" To this I reply, "Of course, nothing in medicine is mathematically certain, but I believe this condition will never return. You are much more likely to meet your end from an automobile accident, atom bomb or even old age!"

Apropos of this discussion is a letter I received from a man whose mother was dying of cancer. By means of a biopsy and x-ray study, hopeless spread (metastases) of cancer into the skull had been found. In fear and trembling the patient and her husband came to my office. That I succeeded in reassuring them and making everyone concerned much happier is evident from the son's letter:

"This is just a pathetically inadequate effort on my part to tell you how beautifully you are handling mother's case, and how grateful my brothers and I are for men like you. I arrived home just as mother and father had come from your office after the x-ray pictures. It was a revelation—the change you worked on them both was wonderful to see. Mother has talked of nothing else all evening—of how relieved she is—and of a completly renewed hope. Again, with many thanks and a lasting appreciation of all you have done for our family."

Sometimes a patient squarely faces the fact that he has a fatal cancer, and he emphatically insists that the diagnosis be kept secret from the family. This may ostensibly be agreed upon, but the doctor and the family must always be in full confidence. It is axiomatic that a doctor must tell the family the diagnosis and, as accurately as he can predict it, the probable duration of the illness. No amount of consideration for the family's feelings permits a doctor to withhold from them the true state of affairs.

There are few occasions in which a physician's skill, understanding and kindness can be of more value and importance, both to the patient and to his family, than when death is inevitable. Fatal illnesses are usually the greatest test of a doctor's patience and sympathy. The time has long passed since one heard the expression: "Old Doctor Smith never lost a patient." Such a reference is actually uncomplimentary, because it stigmatizes the doctor either as dishonest or as so incompetent that no one trusts him with anything but the most minor ailment. When a patient's life is slowly ebbing, and inevitable defeat is looming more and more clearly, then, if ever, do the family and the patient lean upon the doctor for support.

While I believe that one should never admit that defeat is sure, although it seems so, I do not think it is justifiable or fair to the patient or his family, when the end seems close, to give treatments, especially costly blood transfusions, to prolong the life. Only sufficient intravenous fluids should be given to alleviate discomfort from dehydration. And of course the use of narcotics is always indicated for pain in such a case. The family's chief concern is that the patient's suffering is allayed. During such a trying period the physician must expend his time and energy to the important task of bolstering the family's morale. They as well as the patient are suffering, and the physician's duty is to help them all he can.

At this point it is appropriate to comment upon euthanasia, the painless putting to death of some one suffering from what is believed to be an incurable disease, an act to which the dubious term "mercy killing" has been applied. In the present state of civilization, for reasons based upon "the most good to the most people," this type of killing is legally forbidden and is ethically improper. For generations, physicians have done everything in their power to minimize the sufferings of those afflicted with a painful malignant growth. To this end they have decreased pain and avoided efforts which would merely prolong a hopeless existence. To entrust one's fate to a physician of kindly sympathy and highest ethical standards is the best solution of the problem. It seems unfortunate to have euthanasia brought forth as a subject for lay debate, as it is almost impossible for those who are inexperienced in medical matters to evaluate the premises of the argument. To me, freeing a patient of most of his pain by means of drugs is no more reprehensible than eliminating pain during an operation by means of anesthetics. However, to put the power of execution into a doctor's hands is perilous.

In recent years the term "palliative operation" has come to be used with increasing frequency and with a matter-of-fact assurance which would imply that it has a well delimited, generally accepted significance. The words mean the mitigation of a disease process when cure is considered to be impossible. Its indications and its applications to a particular situation may well require soul-searching consideration on the part of the surgeon. A categorical indication for the severance of certain nerves is the presence of an inoperable malignant tumor which is causing intolerable pain. On the other hand, there is seldom any justification for excision of a nonobstructing malignant growth in the stomach which has already spread (metastasized) beyond its primary site. An intermediate situation is presented when the liver is found to contain metastases from the cancer of the colon which is threatening to cause intestinal obstruction, a condition which would be fatal many months before the hepatic involvement would cause death. In such a case, the "palliative" removal of the cancerous mass in the colon would be highly proper.

Some of the most severe strain to which a surgeon is subjected comes, not in the operating room, but during a difficult, prolonged, sometimes fatally ending postoperative course. Such an ordeal may last for days or even weeks, during which time the surgeon must stimulate himself and all those connected with the case to exert maximum energy and thoughtfulness. I can recall many periods of terrific stress. In one case, an embolism of the pulmonary artery simulated for days a leaky duodenal stump following gastric resection, but at the postmortem examination the stump proved to be entirely exonerated. Similarly, in another case, gallstone colic was thought to be a symptom of a leaking duodenal stump after gastric resection. In an especially difficult case, an unsuccessful fight for the life of a patient with necrotizing pancreatitis subsequent to a common duct operation demanded most of our time, thought and strength for a month.

CHAPTER VI

The Surgeon in the Operating Room

FROM the perspective of many years of experience it may be proper to offer some counsel on the general conduct of the surgeon in the operating room. First of all, he should be courteous and businesslike when "booking" an operation, that is, when he calls to reserve the date and time for an operation. He may find that it is impossible to secure a desirable time and will have to take a second choice. This is not the booking clerk's or nurse's fault (unless she is obviously inexperienced), and the surgeon should not argue and try to squeeze his case in the schedule, regardless of causing inconvenience to other surgeons and their teams. If, over a period of time, it appears that the operating room staff is not being utilized to maximum efficiency, usually the matter can be straightened out by a conference between the operating room supervisor and the chief surgeon or the staff operating room committee.

It has long been my belief that the smartest and most efficient service in an operating room is developed by rigid insistence on good technique combined with uniform courtesy. A mature surgeon often forgets how almost completely ignorant of surgical procedures a young intern and/or a young nurse may be. Almost invariably each is trying earnestly, even desperately, to give all the help he can. This spirit can be fully utilized to produce the highest proficiency if simple, courteous, polite instructions are given and if, when possible, an explanation of the purpose of any service requested is patiently made. Development of an enthusiastic *esprit de corps* will evolve a brilliant operating team, each member having pride in his team membership. A surgeon who is a loud, bitingly sarcastic, unjust martinet will never develop this precious team spirit. Despite the fact that the surgeon is working harder and is under much greater strain than anyone else in the operating room, he is not excused from remembering that the others also are working hard and, in fact, may be nearer to the point of exhaustion than he is. The surgeon alone has the great stimulation of initiating and carrying through various manual procedures, so the motivating force is much less strong in the first assistant and practically nonexistent in the "retractor men." I frequently call for momentary rest periods for the entire team, during which the retractor men can relax and exercise their cramped fingers. Exchanging the positions of the second and third assistants to opposite sides of the table may prove restful to them. The surgeon should show his awareness of the necessarily delayed or missed mealtimes of his assistants and try to avoid their becoming excessively fatigued.

I believe that it often helps the partnership in the operating room to make the homely comparison of the surgical personnel and a football team. The surgeon is the "ball carrier," whose performance is relatively easy if the "retractor men" and the first assistant do the proper "blocking" and if they "open up holes in the line." Another measure which contributes to a favorable *esprit de corps* is the "signal system." I saw this system developed to a high degree by my former chief, Dr. Eugene Pool, in New York in 1916. According to this system the surgeon puts out his right hand in the direction of the instrument table and makes one of many different hand signals, which an alert nurse interprets, and she then quickly places the indicated instrument in his hand. Every one on the team learns the signals and develops pride in the smartness with which the system is put into play. This signal system has the merit of minimizing the number of spoken words and hence the number of mouth organisms extruded into the face mask and possibly through it to the operative field.

I believe it is also helpful for the surgeon to address each member of the team by name, for instance referring to an assistant as "Dr. Smith," the term "Doctor" being used as a courtesy. After a resident has worked with me for a year, I usually address him by his first name. The chief nurse is always addressed as "Miss (or Mrs.) ——," even if the surgeon must take a few seconds before the operation to learn what her name is by inquiring of the supervisor.

The great English surgeon Sir Frederick Treves, "surgeon extraordinary to Queen Victoria," is said to have remarked concerning surgeons that a shaking hand offers a slight obstacle by prolonging the duration but not the success of an operation, but that a shaking mind is an insuperable obstacle. As Burrows[24] puts it: "The calm, well-stocked brain is of much more consequence to the operator than the steady hand and wonderful dexterity that appeal to popular imagination."

It is taken for granted that the surgeon starts each operation with all possible knowledge of the problem presented by the case and with the proper knowledge and technical skill for taking care not only of what is likely to be found but whatever may unexpectedly be encountered. The value of all these essentials is diminished, however, if the surgeon does not possess the full measure of that most priceless quality, *equanimity*. This does not mean that he should not be quick and energetic and make decisions promptly. Sir William Osler,[3] in his superb valedictory address entitled "Aequanimitas," delivered at the University of Pennsylvania in 1889, said:

> "In the physician or surgeon no quality takes rank with imperturbability . . . coolness and presence of mind under all circumstances, calmness amid storm, clearness of judgment in moments of great peril, immobility, impassiveness . . . in a true and perfect form, imperturbability is indissolubly associated with a wide experience and with an intimate knowledge of the varied aspects of disease."

Finney[2] urges that the surgeon, in order to cultivate the much desired quality of equanimity, should give careful study and implicit observance in his work to the following fundamental rules of good surgery:

> "Let me emphasize as strongly as I can the advisability, indeed the absolute necessity, for the exercise of unremitting diligence and scrupulous care in the performance of a surgical operation. A large part of good surgery consists in strict attention to detail in everything that concerns the operation: a carefully taken history; a thorough physical examination; the making of a correct diagnosis; the prepara-

tion of the patient mentally as well as physically for the operation; the choice of anesthetist and anesthetic; absolute asepsis; careful and gentle handling of the tissues; absolute hemostasis; avoidance of the devitalization of tissues in the wound by ligation of unnecessarily large masses of tissue or by too tight sutures; the use of the finest silk in suture and ligature material [with certain exceptions. F.C.]; omission of drainage in clean, dry wounds; accurate approximation of wound and skin flaps; physiological rest after operation [compatible with judicious early ambulation. F.C.]; avoidance of too tight dressings and bandages. These are the fundamental laws of good surgery as insisted upon by that master surgeon, Professor William Stewart Halsted, my honored chief for thirty-three years."

Certainly a surgeon's equanimity in the operating room bears a direct relation to the scope of his experience and the frequency with which he has encountered and dealt with unusual findings or happenings. Equanimity is a noble and indispensable quality never to be confused with the pernicious quality of conceited and flippant self-assurance. No matter how many times a surgeon has performed an operation and no matter how simple it has become to him, he must always approach it with maximum care and watchfulness. I have told my residents many times that when a surgeon comes to consider an operation as "easy," his soul is lost. Although some operations are admittedly more difficult than others, it is best for the surgeon (and for his patient) to remember that no operation is really easy. As I review the technical errors I have made in my surgical career, I feel that they happened usually when I thought I was doing something that was easy. When an operation is most difficult, the surgeon is most attentive, careful and watchful, but whenever he feels ultraconfident, his concentration may stray. That is when danger lurks beside him.

The critical tests of a surgeon's equanimity at the operating table come in many forms. Sometimes he meets these tests when fortified by a good night's sleep, but many times the tests come at 3 A.M. after an exhausting day, or near the end of a five-hour operation. It is then that he must draw on his nervous and physical reserves which, it is hoped, he has carefully guarded against depletion due to activities unrelated to his professional work and due to inadequate care of his own health.

The first type of test of equanimity is concerned with the patience and care necessary to complete long, delicate operations, such as an anastomosis deep in the pelvis, or a total gastrectomy.

The second type deals with unanticipated findings, for instance, when the preoperative diagnosis was acute appendicitis but operation reveals carcinoma of the cecum or a perforated duodenal ulcer necessitating a different incision and an operation of much greater magnitude and difficulty. The surgeon must have the mental elasticity and adaptability to adjust himself to every new problem. He must avoid the rigid, stubborn type of thinking which attempts to make inadequate findings fit a predetermined diagnosis, at the expense of failing to make a complete search and actually overlooking the real trouble. I have in mind a surgeon who removed an appendix even though its normal appearance worried him somewhat, but not sufficiently to stimulate him to make a careful search, which would have disclosed the perforated diverticulum of the ascending colon in time to repair it successfully and save the patient's life. A surgeon should never be content with an inadequate explanation of any physical findings, but must search for some other explanation, which is often found.

The third type of test of the surgeon's equanimity is concerned with the unexpected happenings, of infinite variety, such as a loud noise when an instrument pan crashes to the floor or an electric light bulb explodes. The lighting system may fail and require the use of emergency battery lights, with which every operating room should be equipped. During an operation I have seen a nurse slip on a wet floor and fall down, breaking her arm, and I have seen an assistant or a nurse become ill and have to leave the operating room. Occasionally an assistant may make an error, requiring the re-doing of many tedious steps. I have had an anesthetist let my patient get too "light" before a large incision had been secured and cause it to rupture, a mishap which required the repetition of an hour's work.

An unexpected hemorrhage may be a rigorous test of the surgeon's emotional stature. A small artery can shoot a vigorous stream of blood into the surgeon's face (including his eyes and glasses) but can be readily secured. However, a hemorrhage deep in the recesses of the abdomen, where the source is concealed by a rapidly forming lake of blood, is most difficult to control, for instance when a cystic artery of the gallbladder or a renal artery is uncontrolled. An inexperienced and frightened surgeon may plunge a hemostat into the puddle of blood in an effort to grasp the bleeding artery, a procedure that carries the great risk of injury to some adjacent structure. For example, the common bile duct might be injured in the case of hemorrhage from the cystic artery. In such an instance the surgeon should control the bleeding by inserting a finger in the foramen of Winslow and compressing the hepatic ligament until the bleeding point can be accurately located. Most hemorrhages can be retarded or stopped by firm pressure with a warm laparotomy pad. This may be applied for five to twenty minutes and then quickly snatched away, with resultant clear demonstration of the source of the bleeding. In that instant the bleeding point can be seen and grasped with a hemostat. I have used such a pack long enough to send for an extra assistant and keep up the pressure on it until he has scrubbed up for the operation. To me one of the most alarming hemorrhages is that resulting from injury to the portal vein during removal of the gallbladder. In one case in which the hemorrhage was from the portal vein and in another case in which it was from a renal artery, I was able to clamp the bleeding point but was unable to ligate it. In each instance I had to leave the clamp on for a week. Both patients recovered. The hemorrhage from a duodenal ulcer may tax the surgeon's resources; he must work rapidly while massive transfusions are being administered.

In operating upon a patient with intestinal obstruction due to adhesions, the surgeon occasionally opens the intestine inadvertently during the course of the delicate dissection. No blame is attached to this occurrence, but the wound must be patiently repaired, sometimes by time-consuming, painstaking resection.

One of my own most difficult situations comes to mind vividly. This patient was an elderly woman with cancer of the right colon. Her heart was none too good. In fact, before the operation, the anesthetist stated with finality: "You will be able to do only a colostomy." Why he thought an opening in the bowel distal to the cancer would do any good was never explained. Nevertheless, the patient did tolerate most admirably a difficult, three-hour resection of the right colon. Afterward, I went to lunch with my tired team, and then we stopped in at the pathology laboratory to inspect the excised specimen. The head pathologist, Dr. John McCarter, examined it and made the alarming statement that a large piece of the urinary bladder was attached to the specimen. I immediately telephoned the special nurse who was taking care of the patient and was told that urine had been obtained by catheterization. However, her report could not have been correct, as Dr. McCarter's frozen section proved that the tissue in question actually was from the bladder wall. Evidently the cancer had become attached to the bladder, and during the operation some of the bladder wall had been excised along with the tumor. Uncorrected, this situation would have been fatal. So, with heavy heart, I had the little old lady taken back to the operating room that afternoon and opened the abdomen through a new incision. The bladder was "purse-stringed" around a mushroom catheter. This "last ditch" stand was successful, and the patient made a fine recovery. Seven years later she was alive and well, with no sign of recurrence.

Nowadays, cessation of breathing seldom occurs, but during my surgical career I have witnessed a number of these alarming occurrences. The most vivid recollection is that of a fine, sturdy boy, about six years old, who sustained a small laceration in a fall. As he was too frightened to permit sutures with local anesthesia only, a general anesthetic had to be given, unfortunately when the stomach was full. It would have been best to have used no anesthesia, despite the parents' indignant reproaches of cruelty. As I was about to suture the wound, the boy vomited and chunks of meat blocked his windpipe. His pupils dilated, breathing stopped and his color became dusky blue. The nurse anesthetist threw up her hands and cried (helpfully), "He's gone!" The intern and I dropped all sterile precautions, dug the food out of the air passage and kept up artificial respiration until the boy was breathing satisfactorily. I then completed the surgical work, but must confess that while I was doing it the thought kept flashing through my mind of how close I had been to the onerous duty of informing the parents that their boy was dead.

When the heart stops beating (cardiac arrest), the situation is even more dangerous. If the surgeon's hands are in the abdomen, he can massage the heart outside of or through an incision in the diaphragm. Otherwise, he must make an incision in the thoracic wall in order to grasp and massage the heart. There are numerous reported cases of success by both methods, but neither has been successful in my hands in the few instances in which I have used them.

Another strain upon the surgeon's equanimity is to hear, as he is about to close the abdomen or may have completely closed it, the scrub nurse state ominously, "The sponge count is incorrect."

This means that one of the counted pieces of gauze or one of the laparotomy pads is missing and, despite all hunting in floor basins and elsewhere, cannot be found. This is a most trying situation and fortunately is infrequent. The surgeon may feel virtually sure the missing sponge is not in the abdominal cavity, but cold evidence points to the possibility that it may be. The matter must be settled before the patient is taken from the operating room or wakes up from the anesthesia. Usually another search will disclose the missing gauze under a drape sheet or under a towel in a basin.

I recall one instance in which a fourth year medical student, about to leave the operating room for a class, spied a bloody piece of gauze on the operating room floor. Doubtless wishing to do his good deed for that day, he discreetly picked up the object and walked out in the hall. But what to do with it? After some search he found a trash can in a "duty room" at the other end of the hall, where he disposed of the gauze and went happily on his way. Meanwhile, back in the operating room, the surgeon did not dare close the incision, and all of the operating room personnel continued searching until the missing gauze was found.

It is now mandatory that all pieces of gauze introduced into the abdomen contain a small piece of metal-impregnated cardboard which is x-ray opaque. When a piece of gauze cannot be accounted for, a portable x-ray machine is used at the operating table. If it shows that the gauze is not in the abdomen, the surgeon may safely complete the closing of the incision.

Burrows[24] says:

"Another kind of surgical occasion which calls for firmness of character is when at a critical moment during an operation some onlooker intervenes with an ill-timed remark. The effect upon the surgeon may be compared with that exerted upon a sprinter who happens to be jostled by a competitor in a hundred-yard race. Whether he deviates to the right or to the left as a result of the collision will depend upon whether action or reaction is greater; but in either event his balance will be disturbed and his even stride be broken. In the case of the surgeon the disturbance caused will be proportional not only to his mental concentration at the moment, but also to his instability of character."

I have more than once heard some crude remark made by a bystander at an operation with the intention of being humorous, only to find to his dismay that the patient was under local anesthesia and must have heard the remark.

During my more than five thousand major operations, I have always felt conscious of my obligation to instruct those who were helping me. The foremost factor in this instruction is to perform each operation with the maximum skill, care and adequacy possible. The assistants thus learn what I believe to be the proper way to do each particular operation. Despite my own zeal to "carry on," I have tried to be ever mindful that an assistant holding a retractor may not be able to see the area on which I am working or what I am doing. Whenever I think that it is not incompatible with the patient's best interests, I call for a momentary pause and point out the various landmarks and the steps I am taking. This not only saves the assistant from a virtual waste of time but actually, because of the brief respite, makes him a more rested and valuable assistant.

I have always felt in the case of a private patient who engages me to do an operation that there is an unwritten contract or understanding that I do all of it; therefore I almost invariably close even the skin myself and then dictate my operative report and check the immediate postoperative orders. The Board of Regents of the American College of Surgeons in supporting the surgical residency training program is a little sensitive that this domain not overlap that of pernicious "ghost surgery." At their meeting in Cleveland on May 1, 1954, the Board "clarified" an earlier (spring, 1954) definition of ghost surgery by making the following statement:[38]

> "A surgical operation represents a co-operative effort by the responsible surgeon and his assistant. The exact part which each plays during a particular operation may well and frequently does vary. Ghost surgery has been defined by the Regents as that surgery in which the patient is not informed of, or is misled as to, the identity of the operating surgeon. The Board considers it to be a breach of ethics when any patient who has made an agreement with a surgeon is operated upon by another without knowledge and consent of the patient. However, the Board considers it proper for the responsible surgeon to delegate to his assistant the performance of any part of a given operation, provided the surgeon is an active participant throughout the essential part of the operation. The Board of Regents approves the inclusion of all patients in residency training programs."

Myers[39] comments upon the deficiencies in training obtained by preceptorship as contrasted with an approved residency program:

> "If the preceptee attaches himself as an assistant or a partner to the preceptor and hopes to learn surgery on the private patients of the

preceptor, the legal responsibility of the preceptor for the acts of the preceptee must be kept in mind. In a recent malpractice suit in which the plaintiff patient was awarded $200,000 damages from a surgeon and the hospital, the following is an excerpt from the instructions of the judge to the jury: 'An attending physician who has undertaken the care and treatment of a patient cannot assign the performance of an operation or procedure to an assistant which fact is unknown to the patient and escape liability for negligence. . .' "

A few residents are resentful if they are not permitted to put in the skin sutures themselves, but they learn little from doing it and will have more than ample opportunity for this later. When I was chief surgeon at the Evanston Hospital, I acted for many years as the first assistant to the resident or intern in all nonprivate cases in which he was eligible to operate and capable of doing so. Later, as I became more pressed for time, I delegated these teaching tasks to the younger surgeons on the staff. In an excellent editorial on the "Teaching of Surgical Technic," in the March 4, 1954 issue of the *New England Journal of Medicine*, the following question from a report of the New England Surgical Society is quoted: "Can surgeon ethically turn over all or part of an operation on one of his private patients to a member of the resident staff for teaching purposes?" The *Journal* adds:

> "The very fact that the report asks such a question and goes to some pains to answer it indicates that in the minds of the authors the teaching of surgical technic is a serious problem. . . . Any attempt to separate 'surgical technic' from the totality of a surgical operation leads to the concept that a man might be trained to be a good technician while yet a poor surgeon, whereas by any reasonable classification a man who does poorly by his patient at the operating table is a poor exponent of surgical technic and must be regarded as a poor technician no matter how flashy his handling of the knife. . . . There is a deplorable tendency to regard the mere teaching of the surgical operation as something that is below the dignity of an educator, who should be more concerned with psychiatry, social service, biochemistry or physiology. This unfortunate state of mind arises from much too narrow a definition of the technical aspects of surgery. When it is put in its proper reference, and the act of surgery is defined as the surgical operation and everything pertaining to it, it looms as one of the most important, if not the most important, single event in the care of the surgical patient."

For years it has been my practice when doing the more or less routine procedures requiring less concentrated attention, such as closing the abdomen, to quiz my assistants informally. Various hypothetical questions not only revive them mentally and physically but are intended to instruct them by making them think about the answers. Such questions include: "How would you recognize a postoperative hemorrhage from a large branch of the inferior epigastric artery causing a huge hematoma just outside the peritoneum?" "How would you handle a severe wound disruption?" "What would you do if you were the surgeon and these Penrose tubing drains, which we have just placed after a cholecystectomy, were inadvertently pulled out before the dressing was applied?" "What would you do for the first aid of a sucking wound of the chest at the scene of an automobile accident?" I usually let each of the men present give an answer.

CHAPTER VII

Anesthesia

IMPORTANT factors in the patient's safety and the surgeon's free-dom to concentrate his attention on an operation are the skill, attitude and emotional make-up of the anesthetist. Great strides have been made in anesthesiology in the last fifty years, and we have come a long way from the early crude methods. Forty years ago, an intern might be summoned in haste to give his first anes-thetic without previous instructions because the operating room was shorthanded. This happened to me in 1915, the surgeon merely saying that he would advise me how much ether to pour on. After a long struggle with a cyanotic short-necked, fat man whose false teeth, as I afterwards learned, were bumping around in his throat, I finally completed the anesthesia, and the patient miraculously survived.

Most of the best early anesthetists were women, chiefly nurses, but a few were doctors, and they were always gentle and consid-erate. Today some states permit anesthetics to be given only by a doctor of medicine.

Today, anesthesiology is a definite, distinct specialty and has its Board of Certification, one of the nineteen specialty boards. Before becoming eligible to take the examinations for board certification, an applicant must, among other things, "submit proof to the Board that he has limited his practice to Anesthesiology as a specialty for five calendar years, of which at least two have been in formal training approved by the Board. He must be a member in good standing of the American Society of Anesthesiologists, Inc." He must also "prove to the satisfaction of the Board by such written, survey, oral and practical examinations as the Board may prescribe that he is qualified to practice Anesthesiology; and . . . . personally prepare such case history abstracts of personally conducted procedures pertaining to Anesthesiology as the Board may specify." The written examinations include "anatomy, chemistry, physics, pharmacology, pathology and physiology." The fee is $125.00.

Many young doctors are attracted to anesthesiology as a specialty because there is usually more regularity of hours and more financial security after one has become established. Up until recently, and in some situations this system still obtains, the anesthetist was salaried by the hospital, and his services were paid for by the patient when he settled his hospital bill, included under the subheading "charge for the operating room" or "charge for anesthesia." The current, widely prevalent practice is for the anesthetist to send his own separate bill directly to each patient. Furthermore, the patient must pay this bill, although he has not personally selected his anesthetist. Indeed, the surgeon also usually has no voice in the matter, but must accept whoever is assigned him and is expected to tell the patient that the anesthetist's bill, whatever it may be, is proper. In general, however, this system is an improvement, as it develops competition among anesthetists to give the best service possible and insures a more careful preoperative scrutiny of the patient by the anesthetist and more attentive after-care.

Richard K. Gilchrist[40] recently said:

> "The surgeon is very willing in teaching institutions to say, 'We are now approaching a danger point, and unfortunately we have had something happen,' but in my experience it is almost impossible to get the anesthetist in the teaching institution to say as the operation progresses and you have residents and students present, 'The patient's condition is this; the preoperative medication is this; the drugs given to this point are these; and we will now add this, that and the other. We will cooperate.' They are very reluctant to do so."

Koontz[41] says: "Certainly the anesthetist should do nothing to the patient to start violent struggling without discussing the matter with the surgeon first. . . . In general, it should never be lost sight of that surgical anesthesia is an adjunct to surgery and not an end in itself." Potts[42] has well said that "a few" physician-anesthesiologists can justify their long period of training "only by doing unusual things for the routine operation when a simple method would be safer."

Of course, the picture is not always as gloomy as this. I have known many anesthetists for whom I have the highest regard and whose loyalty to me was unquestioned. During an operation I needed only exchange a glance with the anesthetist in order to know my patient's condition. His look or a few quiet words have often given me the added encouragement I needed to go more slowly and more painstakingly. When such an anesthetist looked grave, I knew he was sincere in warning me to hasten the operation in every way possible. Some other type of anesthetist might give the same warning, but being largely self-centered he is motivated more by what someone might say of the manner of the anesthetic's administration than by team spirit to help the surgeon through a difficult period.

An admirable statement of the optimum surgeon-anesthetist rapport has been made by Cole and Sadove[43]:

"Efficiency of operative care of the patient is not possible without complete cooperation between the surgeon and anesthesiologist. The added responsibilities acquired during the past decade or two by the anesthesiologist have considerably changed the role of the anesthesiologist in the operative care of the patient. The anesthesiologist's knowledge of such subjects as pharmacology and physiology have made him very helpful to the surgeon in the care of the patient. There are so many variable factors in hospitals throughout the country that the responsibilities of the surgeon and anesthesiologist cannot be defined dogmatically. Many of these functions will have to be worked out according to circumstances; however, certain of them are rather obvious. For example, the surgeon and anesthesiologist should consult preoperatively, and, after the anesthesiologist has had opportunity to examine the patient and his chart, the surgeon should inform the anesthesiologist of the type of operation planned and the anesthesiologist should inform the surgeon of the type of anesthetic he contemplates using. The anesthesiologist should inform the surgeon promptly of any change in the patient's condition during the operation. Likewise, the surgeon should inform the anesthesiologist immediately of any change in the operative plan. The surgeon expects the anesthesiologist to keep constant watch over the patient's condition, and the anesthesiologist expects the surgeon to perform the operation with the least amount of trauma and minimal blood loss. The operation is no place for prejudice or anger. We must remember at all times that the welfare of the patient is the paramount issue during an operation. Complete cooperation will result in maximal efficiency."

To get the training prerequisite to the taking of the examinations for Board certification in anesthesia, physicians naturally try to obtain residencies in anesthesia in institutions where they will get the most experience and instruction. We do not know just what the Anesthesia Board specifies when it requires the candidate for examination to "personally prepare such case history abstracts of personally conducted procedures." Certainly the candidate will naturally wish to submit the largest number of reports on spinal anesthesias, intratracheal intubations, etc., that he can. There may be pressure upon him or on the chief anesthetist to employ a more complicated procedure when a simpler one would be better.

I have felt strongly about my responsibility for the unconscious patient in the operating room. The patient or his family cannot protect his interests there, and they rely upon me to do it. If a new intern is unfortunate enough to have to puncture the patient's arm four or five times to find a vein, one is not surprised to hear a patient loudly protest and a call for someone who is not "practicing" on him. Happily the patient in the operating room cannot see the resident in anesthesia getting the material for his "personally conducted procedures" in support of his application for Board certification. It is the surgeon who must "explain" to his patient after an operation why he has a sore throat that may be more annoying than the pain of the incision. The solution of this difficult problem lies in a combination of factors: a chief anesthetist with time to supervise and a conscience that will put the patient's interest ahead of the resident's rate of progress and his own teaching prestige, the use of more nurse anesthetists in simple cases, and the forthrightness on the part of surgeons to defend their patients' interests in hospital executive circles.

Beecher and Todd[44] have recently published an important contribution entitled "A Study of the Deaths Associated with Anesthesia and Surgery." They made a study of *all deaths* attributable to anesthesia in 599,548 operations at ten participating university hospitals from January 1, 1948, to December 31, 1952. Twenty-one physicians and eleven secretaries worked on this report continuously for five years. The results have been a revelation. It used to be said, some forty years ago, that the death rate from ether was about 1 in 20,000. With the improvements and discoveries of anesthesia, surgeons have come to feel that modern anesthesiology is really much safer than it was a generation ago. However, it is only a courageous and laborious study, such as that of Beecher and Todd, which proves that the reverse is true: They say:

> "Data are presented to show that death from anesthesia is of sufficient magnitude to constitute a public health problem. Anesthesia kills several times as many citizens each year out of the total population of the country as does poliomyelitis. Consideration of the millions of dollars rightly spent in attacking poliomyelitis and the next to nothing, comparatively, spent in anesthesia research makes clear an urgent need." [Of course, during the period of this study, many more deaths from poliomyelitis occurred than, happily, occur now, with the protection of the Salk vaccine. F. C.]

Beecher and Todd found that: 1. "Inhalation anesthesia is by far the single most important technic; but the use of intravenous anesthesia has doubled in the period of study, while the use of the spinal technic has declined somewhat. It accounts, surprisingly, for less than 9 per cent of the cases." 2. "The use of ether as a primary agent is steadily increasing, while the use of cyclopropane is not rising." 3. "When muscle relaxants (curare) were used the 'anesthesia death rate increases nearly six-fold.'" 4. The over-all anesthesia death rate, that is, primary anesthesia death and death where anesthesia was described as an important contributory cause of death, was 1:1560, which is quite different from 1:20,000. 5. A fifth of the anesthetics were administered by nurses. 6. Forty per cent of anesthetics were administered by anesthesia residents. 7. Fifty-nine per cent of the "non-curare deaths" and 63 per cent of the "curare deaths" were at the hands of residents in anesthesia. 8. Eighteen per cent of the "non-curare deaths" and 19 per cent of the "curare deaths" were at the hands of nurse anesthetists.

CHAPTER VIII

Surgical Pitfalls

N<small>O ONE</small> who enters into the specialty of surgery should delude himself into thinking that he will never make an error. In a long surgical career, every surgeon looks back upon cases in which he wishes that he had done differently. Perhaps, here and there, a different step or procedure might have spelled the difference between life and death. He can only prepare himself most fully and intensely and operate with greatest care, coolness and judgment.

No human being can be free from error, but it must be one's constant effort to reduce these errors to the minimum. A surgeon's error may be incalculably costly, since a human life is at stake.

Each day the surgeon must alert himself continually to the possibility of error of judgment or of technique and never think of any decision or procedure as "easy." In the determination of an error, postmortem examination is of prime importance. It is one of the great foundation stones of medical progress. If a surgeon makes an error, he must bear it with dignity and courage and not "fold up." He knows that he must carry on, that it has taken a long time for him to be "manufactured" and that his services must be available to those who need them—services that after an error has been made will be more valuable and more skilled, rather than less so.

Should the surgeon fall into the reprehensible attitude of feeling sorry for himself, he should be enheartened by comparing his responsibilities with those of military leaders. A surgeon's error may cost one life, but a general's error may send hundreds of thousands of fine young men to their death. "Someone had blundered . . .

Theirs not to reason why, Theirs but to do and die." And the states-man's error in judgment or the ruler's need to strengthen his popu-larity may plunge whole nations into catastrophe. I think that most people realize that no surgeon can be absolutely infallible. All that they want are his utmost efforts and deepest thought.

That no one, no matter how skilled and conscientious, is immune to error is discussed by J. M. T. Finney.[2] He tells how even Sir William Osler failed to recognize acute appendicitis in a Johns Hopkins nurse, despite Finney's warnings, and her appendix per-forated and peritonitis developed. After a stormy session on the "Ochsner Treatment" and drainage of recurrent pelvic abscesses, the patient finally recovered. Finney says:

> "Mistakes are not confined to people of low intelligence or of little experience, although unquestionably they are far more common in those classes. It is the wise man who benefits by his errors, and often one learns more from his mistakes than from his successes. Although it is only natural that one does not want to herald widely one's misdeeds, still it is well in all humility to report them in order that others may profit by such mistakes and so avoid as far as possible their repetition in the future. A thorough study of a mistake in order to satisfy oneself, if possible, as to just how it occurred and how it could have been avoided, may prove helpful."

In 1922, Harold Burrows, of Portsmouth, England, published a volume entitled "Mistakes and Accidents of Surgery." In his preface he said:

> "Sea captains of old sailed in waters that were uncharted. Their guides were nebulous and doubtful; their dangers great. The steep coast, the gently shelving shore—such poor marks as these—inter-preted by them, vaguely and with much hazard, what now is told truly and surely in the chart house. The surgeon of today is like the sailor of a past age. He, too, is embarked upon oceans that are unmapped and wide. Forever, and with much labour, feeling his way with the lead, as it were, he is beset with incessant troubles. Innumerable are the surgical disasters with which he is menaced, unnoticed or un-recorded are their causes, unavoidable their repetition. My aim has been to make a commencement of better things by locating some of the danger points in the universe of surgery. The charting I have ac-complished is rough and imperfect—almost absurd may be—like the early maps of the world in its simplicity and crudity. Nevertheless, there is value in the ill-shapen beginnings of a thing, for we know that all the complex tracery of completion will come eventually as the gift of time."

In less than three years a second edition of Burrow's book was called for, and in the preface of this new edition he remarks:

"The first edition of this book fell into the hands of the lay press. Sensational copy could be extracted by unscrupulous journalists, and so material, which had been intended for medical men alone, was exploited and misrepresented in order to amuse the public. Therefore, in issuing a second, enlarged and amended edition, it has been thought well to change the title from 'Mistakes and Accidents of Surgery' to 'Pitfalls of Surgery,' and it is hoped that any prejudice or annoyance that was unwittingly created by the former may not be sustained. . . . Textbooks and teachers have been so much concerned with constructive information that relatively little has been said about this subject of the difficulties and dangers of surgery. A minor volume devoted to these matters may therefore be a useful supplement to the major works upon which the surgeon's confidence has been nourished." [The author asks] "to be pardoned for any appearance of pomposity, and assures the reader that many years of labour have taken away all the plumes of pride which once as a young man he possessed and fondly flourished."

While Burrow's book is now somewhat out of date, it still contains much sound advice. He groups surgical errors under four main headings: ignorance, carelessness, misjudgment and defective technique. In the more than five hundred pages of his valuable book are startling and instructive examples of these various errors. He sagely observes:

"We learn by personal experience. To utilize the experience of our colleagues forever is difficult. And yet life is short—is in fact too brief to yield us all that ample knowledge founded upon direct observation which we properly prefer to any second-hand lesson which has been collected by brains other than our own."

The surgeon's energy and fixity of purpose in the unpleasant task of obtaining permission for an autopsy from a grief-stricken and uncomprehending family is an index of sincerity of his search for his errors and his willingness to impart the valuable lesson to other surgeons and thus to benefit other patients. The surgeon who is lukewarm or cold in his efforts to secure necropsies on patients who die after he has operated upon them naturally arouses some suspicion that he is fearful that an error may be revealed. A very fair index of the grade of surgery at a given hospital is the percentage of deaths which come to a postmortem examination. At

Evanston Hospital we have always been proud that the percentage is in the eighties.

The surgeon's conscience may become a battleground between the instinct of self-protection and the necessity for determining the cause of an error, not only for his own identification but for the instruction of others. I have had to get up at midnight and go to the hospital in order to persuade the anguished widow of a patient on whom I had operated to give permission for a postmortem examination. She had become surrounded by a number of suddenly important and, in part, hostile advisers who constantly and loudly interfered.

Every surgeon will find it advisable to carry "physician's liability insurance," for protection in possible "malpractice" suits. One of the leading insurance companies in this field suggests to its policy holders, among other things, that they "make no statements, promises, or take any action which may amount to an admission of liability on your part. . . . In the event of a death under circumstances which may give rise to a claim or suit covered by your policy, report to the company before attending autopsy or inquest." Certainly it is contrary to the advice of insurance companies to admit to a family any technical error which is disclosed at necropsy, but I have not regretted doing so in a single instance. It is to one's colleagues, however, that errors should particularly be explained in order to help prevent their repetition.

In his excellent article on "Medicine and the Law," Regan[36] estimated that 50 to 80 per cent of all malpractice suits would be eliminated if destructive criticism by other physicians could be stopped. He also said:

> "A charge of malpractice is not warranted even by the fact that (the physician) made a mistake in diagnosis or was guilty of an error of judgment, that he might have employed other medicines or used other methods of treatment, that expert witnesses testify that they themselves would have employed a different method or that a bad result followed instead of a satisfactory one. Experience has taught that the most careful attention to the dictates of good medical practice is not sufficient to ward off the unjust claim and that no physician is immune. The likelihood of being sued for malpractice must now be regarded as a definite occupational hazard for the practicing physician. *Caveat medicus!* . . . A patient who has a friendly feeling for the physician and who believes that everything possible has been done for him is not likely to sue for malpractice, even when the result is bad."

Regan stressed the importance of taking x-rays in cases of fracture or suspected fracture, undertaking only such procedures as one is qualified to perform, the employment of consultants in serious or fatal cases, keeping "ideal" records in all cases, obtaining written consent for an operation and approval by special hospital staff committee or reputable consultant before terminating a pregnancy, and the danger of telephoning a prescription.

In a recent issue of the *Bulletin of the American College of Surgeons*[45] appears the following statement:

> "In recent years, the number of malpractice claims has increased fantastically, and, today, approximately 5,000 cases are reported each year—or one case for every 35 doctors in private practice. In some states, the rate is even higher, with as many as one doctor in 12 being involved. Statistics on the subject are not precise, but one authority estimates that the number of malpractice suits has increased twentyfold since World War II.
>
> "Moreover, judgments have soared along with claims, and it is not uncommon today for juries to award $100,000 to a patient they decide has been damaged by his doctor's negligence, carelessness or bad judgment.
>
> "Of course, insurance losses and rates have kept pace with the increases in claims and judgments. In one state alone, two companies reported losses aggregating $3 million since the war. The average cost per malpractice claim to another large company has increased five times since 1941.
>
> "During these years of mounting malpractice claims, the law hasn't changed, and standards of medical and surgical practice have been constantly improved. . . . 'The blunt truth is that the majority of all malpractice suits filed are without merit,' said the late Dr. Louis J. Regan of Los Angeles, who was one of the nation's foremost authorities on forensic medicine. . . . More than half the malpractice suits filed today involve physicians and surgeons who are above the median of their respective groups in skill, experience and professional standing, Dr. Regan stated. 'The bringing of a malpractice action does not even suggest that the claim has merit, for any patient may bring such an action against any physician who has attended him professionally,' he added."

In 1940 a volume of over 700 pages was published entitled *Foreign Bodies Left in the Abdomen,* by H. S. Crossen and D. F. Crossen.[46] The work was undertaken "to emphasize to surgeons the danger of occurrence of the serious accident of leaving a foreign body in the abdominal cavity, to work out the best plan of treatment for various types of such cases, to call attention to the difficulties of avoiding such accident under the many stresses of abdominal work, and to arouse interest in the serious study of the problem of prevention." It makes solemn and valuable reading to study their analysis of 250 reported instances in which a sponge was left in the abdomen and of 86 cases involving a forceps, a part of an instrument, a needle or a drain. Court actions in 108 cases are analyzed. The book includes over 900 references. Foreign bodies have been left not only in the abdominal cavity but in all of the numerous types of surgical wounds. A small gauze sponge may be left under a scalp flap or in a wound of an extremity. An entire needle or a fragment of a needle may be lost in a wound.

Operating on the wrong side is always a menace. Thirty years ago Rutherford Morrison[47] said:

"It seems almost incredible to any but surgeons in a busy hospital that such a horrible mistake was possible. I have seen the wrong side operated upon for inguinal hernia, the wrong kidney explored, the wrong knee joint opened. A house-surgeon of my own amputated the left ring finger of a woman instead of her right. He would have saved himself and the patient much pain and regret and the hospital compensation money if he had remembered my rule: *Always* mark with a cross, before the patient is anesthetized, the side of the body to be operated upon."

Operating on the wrong eye is an especially cruel tragedy. I am thankful that I have never had the misfortune to operate upon the wrong side of a patient's body, but I know of two cases of inguinal hernia in which this happened. I also know of an instance in which the surgeon noticed, when the patient coughed during the induction of anesthesia, that there was a hernia on both sides, instead of just on the one side that had been found at the office examination, and repaired both hernias. The patient, a lawyer, later sued the surgeon for doing more than had been contracted for, but lost his suit.

In view of the fact that when a patient with hernia is unconscious on the operating table it is usually impossible to tell from inspection which side requires operation, the surgeon should always write down which side is involved at the time of the first examination and, as an added precaution, should always ask the patient again in the operating room before the anesthetic is started. In addition, the intern should write this information in the chart, and it is always helpful for the anesthetist also to ask. It is valuable to have the intern mark the proper side with indelible ink or dye when he makes his examination the night before the operation. Extreme care should be taken to avoid confusing language, such as: "Is the left side the right side?" Better: "Is the left side the one needing operation?"

Regarding malpractice suits, the following observations are given in the *Bulletin of the American College of Surgeons*[48]:

> "Careful attention to detail, supervision of personnel in the operating room and on nursing floors, and insistence of completing records and carrying out procedures 'according to the book' will also protect the surgeon against liability. In a New York case not long ago, two private patients, both children, were brought to the operating room floor at the same time. One was scheduled for tonsillectomy, the other for circumcision; both surgeons were on the floor, preparing for the operations.
>
> "At this point, carelessness instead of scrupulous attention to details of operating floor procedure took over, and the children were switched. The child that was to have had a tonsillectomy was circumcised, and the one scheduled for circumcision had the tonsillectomy.
>
> "Later, it developed that instead of following the proper procedure for identifying the patient, one of the surgeons had simply asked the child as he was being wheeled into the anesthetizing area, 'Are you Fred?' and the child answered, 'Yes.'
>
> "Questioned about this, the child remembered that the doctor had spoken to him, but thought he had asked, 'Are you afraid?'
>
> "While this case did result in a lawsuit against one of the surgeons, it was not as serious as some cases of misidentification—such as the classic case in a Chicago hospital, in which a limb was amputated from the wrong patient, or the Michigan case a few years ago in which a woman who was taken to the hospital for treatment of an infected finger wound up in the operating room getting a cholecystectomy.
>
> "In addition to prudence and scrupulous care in the selection and training of employees, record keeping and in actual procedures, there are some special problems in which the malpractice hazard is such that the wise surgeon is well advised to take special precautions in advance of operation. Thus, for example, in all cases of surgery of the head and neck, or the chest, it is advisable to have a preoperative x-ray examination of the jaw to avoid the possibility that the patient may claim later that the operation resulted in damage to the mouth or teeth. The claim that teeth have been damaged by anesthetic equipment, bronchoscope, laryngoscope, or surgical instruments is a frequent one following surgery of the head, mouth or neck, so it is also wise to make a careful examination of the teeth before operation, and see that a description of their condition is inserted in the record, for defense in case of suit."

The following statement appears in another article:[45]

"Studies made by the insurance company that is underwriting the Professional Liability Insurance Program of the American College of Surgeons have identified the following circumstances as substantial causes for professional liability or malpractice actions against surgeons:

"1. Hasty or inconsiderate treatment resulting in poor patient-physician relationship.

"2. Criticism by one physician or surgeon of another's methods or results.

"3. Failure to call in well qualified consultants promptly when surgeon or patient is dissatisfied with progress.

"4. Permitting patient to become overoptimistic about outcome of treatment.

"5. Failure to maintain complete records of history, findings, treatment and operation.

"6. Failure to obtain proper written consent to perform operations.

"7. Failure to instruct and supervise office or hospital assistants properly as to their responsibilities and conduct.

"8. Failure to see that office and hospital equipment and supplies are adequate and maintained in perfect condition.

"9. Patient's dissatisfaction with amount of bill, and surgeon's failure to discuss finances in advance of operation.

"10. Failure to notify insurer or attorney of incidents that might result in malpractice suits."

About 1935 it became apparent to the leading surgical clinics in the United States that silk was, generally speaking, superior to catgut for suture material. I began to use it routinely except in cases in which there was frank pus, as in a ruptured appendix, because it makes a strong wound repair and less reaction occurs around silk than around catgut. Of course, if infection develops in a wound, silk knots or even long pieces of silk may be extruded. On one or two occasions I was obliged to do a minor operation to remove a silk strand that was maintaining an annoying discharging sinus. Of course a catgut knot also may be extruded if infection occurs before the catgut has dissolved. Almost every patient good-humoredly accepts a silk knot extrusion as only a minor complication. One man who went to Florida for his convalescence sent me a picture postal card with the statement: "There is a little present for you under the postage stamp." When the stamp was peeled off, a tiny knot of fine silk was disclosed. One letter from a patient inviting us to be house guests in Florida included the comment that "a stitch abscess delayed the healing of the incision somewhat."

One grateful lady patient sent me a card to which was attached a small piece of silk with the following note: "Dr. Christopher— You planted this in July 1947. It bloomed Easter Sunday 1950. No storage charges."

One of the research workers at Abbott Laboratories, on whom I had done a cholecystectomy, had to come into the office because of persistent draining sinuses, from which I removed silk knots with a small artery forceps. He wrote: "Enclosed is a check to cover the bill for your recent fishing expedition. Your superior angling technique and amazing catch have yielded excellent results. Both sinuses were completely healed within a week. Although I am likely to arouse some speculation among observers as to whether I am the possessor of three umbilici, I think I shall be able to expose my midriff at the beach this summer with little embarrassment."

It was because of one of these silk knots that the only suit for malpractice against me was instituted. This was after over thirty years of active surgical practice and the performing of over 5,200 major operations. Some years after I had operated on a man for acute appendicitis, his eleven-year-old son suffered a severe attack of appendicitis, and at night I removed an unruptured but gangrenous appendix, probably saving his life. Immediately thereafter a wound abscess complicated the recovery, but responded to drainage. Four years later, when the boy was on his high school wrestling team and had driven his car to California, a swelling developed which a surgeon judged to be due to an incarcerated hernia. However, incision disclosed an abscess with some silk knots in the pus. When the surgeon reported this finding to the boy's family, they started suit against me (in 1953), their attorney alleging that my unskillful treatment had been very harmful to the boy and had probably impaired his future earning power. However, after the abscess healed, the boy was soon playing baseball. The suit never came to trial. Early in 1955, the attorneys for the medical liability company were successful in securing from the plaintiff a release in both Superior and Probate courts, and the lawsuit was dismissed.

A physician must never practice without the protection of medical liability insurance. The amount of insurance to carry and the company in which to carry it will have to be decided by the individual and deserves study and inquiry. The amounts and the companies vary in different parts of the country. (See also the chapter on Personal Injury Litigation.)

About a dozen times I have operated upon children after making a preoperative diagnosis of acute appendicitis only to find at operation that the symptoms were due to inflammation of the intestinal lymph nodes (mesenteric lymphadenitis), a condition which would not have required operation, as it would have subsided spontaneously. Were the question to be raised, "Was the operation necessary?" the answer would be decidedly affirmative, for without operation, the correct diagnosis could not have been made and thus the peril of acute appendicitis could not have been eliminated. In each case I have told the parents just what I found and have never been reproached, as they have known that I was only safeguarding their child's welfare; moreover, since the innocent appendix had been removed, they did not have any fear of appendicitis in the future.

A surgeon must never promise a cure *before* operating. But *after* an operation he may tell his patient, in order to encourage him, that he is cured, taking care to inform the family as definitely as possible of the probability of cure.

I have tried to impress on interns, residents and younger surgeons any mistakes I have made, in the hope that they may not only avoid those same mistakes and be on the alert to avoid others, but, moreover, that they may acquire such a constructive attitude of mind that they, in turn, will pass on to succeeding generations the lessons so painfully learned.

CHAPTER IX

Surgical Teaching

I HAVE always been interested in the teaching of medical students, or, as it might better be called, the manufacture of doctors to take care of sick people. While some graduates in medicine enter into special lines of research, administration, and so forth, the great majority spread out over the country to perform the necessary task of caring for the ill. During my thirty-five years of teaching experience, my ideas on this type of instruction have undergone a gradual evolution, leading me to certain conclusions.

My first experience with medical teaching was, naturally, from the student's viewpoint at Johns Hopkins. There from 1911 to 1915 I became imbued somewhat with the Hopkins spirit. It was assumed by the faculty that the students were eager to learn and that the faculty's province was to pour out their knowledge for receptive students. There was never the slightest feeling of "policing" the students or of making them study. If a student did not care to study, that was simply his loss and no one else cared. In fact, as I have said before, in Anatomy under Dr. Franklin P. Mall the requirements for an opportunity to learn were simply "a barn and a stiff." In anatomy no quiz was ever given; there was only a final oral examination as a mechanism by which undesirable students could be eliminated. Although this plan was based on the assumption that the college graduate is a mature and thoughtful individual, I think the idea was carried a little too far at that time at Hopkins.

In the Chicago medical schools, however, it was assumed that the applicants earnestly desired to study, but no chances were taken. The students jolly well had to study, and the degree and intensity of their efforts were frequently appraised by means of tests and examinations, with many gradings. In the end a very satisfactory doctor was manufactured.

Over the years my ideas on medical teaching have been somewhat modified. I have had considerable experience in teaching and observing the effects of instruction upon medical students and young graduates. A new crop of doctors must be produced annually to care for the nation's sick. The present system in medical schools is certainly a vast improvement over the days when Flexner wrote his shattering report, but I feel sure that there is room for much improvement. Perhaps most of the goals are impossible of achievement, but their consideration may be of value.

The first area of improvement is in exposing high school and college students to an accurate presentation of the lifework of a physician; what steps are necessary for preparation; what qualities make for success in the various fields of medical endeavor; what are the costs in time and money and energy for qualifying; what are the satisfactions and spiritual rewards of a successful physician, and what are his possible average financial rewards; what are the necessary health requirements to start with; when is the optimum time for the student to marry; what are the possible disappointments and irritations of medical practice? The average high school student has been making his conclusions on the basis of immature and incomplete premises, as discussed in the opening chapter.

The use of young instructors in medical school is an absolute necessity, but I cannot remember ever receiving great inspiration from them. The young instructors in the clinical branches are often quite inexperienced in the subjects they teach. I believe that these young men would be much better teachers if they were paid small salaries, as is done in law and dental schools, rather than being "rewarded by the prestige of association with a university."

I am inclined to think that the effort to avoid the evils of formal didactic lectures of a generation ago has made the pendulum swing too far in the direction of getting the students in contact with patients. A third year student's time is better spent in studying books, the written words of the masters, than in putting on a white coat and in a group of six or more staring at an embarrassed patient. Of course, the student must learn early, probably in the third year rather than the second, the elements of physical diagnosis, inspection, palpation, percussion and auscultation, but this is best done, as it is at Cook County Hospital in Chicago, in groups not larger than four each, and on free patients only. I do not believe these students can be or should be taught on private patients in a community hospital, although the increase in the various hospitalization and insurance plans is steadily decreasing the number of "free patients," and use of "private patients" for teaching material may be necessary.

Not uncommonly the heads of departments in a medical school have won their positions by pre-eminence in research and/or practice in relatively narrow fields. Many have never engaged in general practice, and when they try to teach the proper way to handle patients, "just as general practitioners do," their instruction is based only on what they imagine is common practice. I certainly do not approve of the practice, sometimes employed by heads of departments, of soliciting from students their anonymous opinions as to the quality of teaching given by their instructors. The heads of the departments themselves are better qualified than the students to form such opinions. Moreover, instructors, when aware of this type of popularity contest, tend to supply entertainment rather than education.

The cornerstones of the acquisition of knowledge by the medical student are textbooks and medical journals. These can often be vivified by a gifted professor, but they can never be supplanted by him. All through a physician's career he will have to think for himself, and his thinking must be based on an intimate knowledge of medical facts as nearly as they can be determined at the time.

I have always felt that my best teaching was to clerks, interns and residents in the hospital, with one, two or possibly three at a time working with me at operations. On daily rounds we would spend time discussing together the strategy of treatment in critical cases, examining patients and letting them hear me converse with patients and their relatives, using words which years of experience have taught me will be of help and comfort. Often I have told these young men that, as it has been in my own case, so it will be with them, an instructive case may seem to have been forgotten for years only to be pulled out of a hidden pigeonhole of the mind when a current situation creates a demand for it.

I have watched with interest and pride the successful careers of scores of young men, and it is a great satisfaction to me to hear from them and to feel that I have been of help to them. Every teacher of medicine receives letters of gratitude from former students, so the following quotations are in no sense singular to me. Even though I do not deserve the praise, these remarks at least delineate what a surgical teacher should try to accomplish.

After helping an applicant win a position at the Mayo Clinic, I received a letter in which he said:

> "My fellowship at the Mayo Clinic begins in a few days, and I want you to know how much I appreciate all that you have done for me. As busy as you have been, you were always able to find time to help me. These few lines are inadequate to express my thanks, but if anyone has done you a great favor, which you found impossible to repay, you will understand how grateful I am to you."

Another letter contained the following:

> "I would like to take this opportunity to express my sincerest thanks for the most enjoyable residency. I find it most difficult to express my gratefulness to you for your teachings and opinions especially when things appeared gloomy, for your untiring patience with me in your efforts to instill some of the principles of surgery. I feel that I have not only gained in the principles of the practice of surgery but in the practice of the art of surgery, which is unfortunately available to only a few of the younger men in our profession."

The following letter was signed by two interns: "This is but a brief note and sent in an attempt to express our appreciation for your kindness in inviting us to your home for dinner. . . . We were quite thrilled and felt highly honored."

During World War II I kept up a correspondence with many of my former clerks, interns, residents and associates who had joined the armed services. Their letters came from all parts of the United States, Alaska, the Pacific, Australia, Burma, the Middle East and Europe. I have saved nearly two hundred of these letters, of which about a third were "V-Mail," and an analysis provides material for a detailed and intimate description of the care of the wounded and life in isolated camps, hospitals and ships. Several examples of G.I. V-mail Christmas cards are interesting. Many of the letters contained comments of personal interest. One V-mail letter, which I later learned was written at Fenton Field, ninety miles south of Darwin, Australia, said: "I was very proud the other day when we opened up the library that was supplied us. There are 19 volumes covering the field of medicine and surgery, and, sure enough, the surgery textbook was 'A Textbook of Surgery' by Christopher. The fellows kidded me a little, saying that I could now refer them to the book instead of giving a discourse on how Dr. Christopher would do it."

Another letter read: "You have no idea how much I have enjoyed working with you and how much I have appreciated your instruction." In thanking me for some Christmas presents of salted nuts and candy: "The tin containers really have the vicious little red ants buffaloed. . . . One of the majors at division headquarters made a statement that you'll appreciate, remembering your army days, and which I thought was pretty good. He said that one sure way of beating the Japs would be to give them all the paper work we have to do."

From an officer in the Amphibious Force of the Navy:

"Since I last wrote you, I've been on the move almost continuously. Adventures of all sorts seem to come my way and the future looks very promising, too. We have passed thru a beauty of a storm; as I write this we are still playing roller coaster and a few of the more sea-sick sailors are poking their heads out of their bunks for the first time in several days. As luck would have it, my immunity to seasickness is apparently very good and that alone is the greatest blessing on these small landing craft. Many ex-destroyer sailors turn up their toes after 24 hours on these little 'bouncing bedpans.' "

The following letter was dated 29 April 1945 and contained such interesting on-the-spot accounts that several sections must be quoted:

"We only dallied a short time at Eniwetok and then went on to Saipan. . . . The Army and the Seabees are as usual busy moving mountains and everything else in their way preparatory to making military establishments. We saw the huge bases for the B-29's and watched them leave and return from their raids on Japan. It is a thrill to see those huge babies whiz down the runway and slowly take the air. They are magnificent machines and are certainly Lord and Master of the Pacific air. . . . From there we went to Iwo Jima and our first baptism of fire. The trip up there was pretty uneventful considering the fact that we expected to be pretty well worked over by the Nip air force. They never showed up, much to our relief, and so we enjoyed perfect weather and ate like kings. Iwo is old stuff to you now, but it will never be forgotten on this ship. From the night during which we approached until we left, it was a most unusual experience. The first big guns that I saw firing in the distance, I thought were thunderstorms. We got into position for the assault undercover of the early morning darkness, and as dawn came you could see hundreds of ships all about in every direction. We were backed up by some real muscle, which eased off everyone's tension a great deal. We had all seen the Intelligence maps of the islands and, as predicted, it was just about glutted with guns. Just before the hour set for the landings, everything grew silent, not even a machine gun popped off, and I think the stillness as we crept up toward the island was the worst part of it all. Suddenly, all Hell broke loose, as the newspapers say, and the show was on. We got fired at quite a bit, but for some reason the Jap artillery in our sector had a hard time getting lateral bearings on us, the shells would start walking up on us and then suddenly no more would come. We figured that they were in caves and the cave side limited their field of fire. So by keeping on the move we emerged unscathed, but pretty well worn out after the first day was over.

CHAPTER X

Surgical Writing

THE writing of medical papers for publication or for delivery before a medical society is usually commendable. Certainly it is not a vice and may even be a virtue. It benefits chiefly the writer, because more than average study of one particular subject is involved. Albert Einstein,[49] with the apology that "A serious-minded man enjoys a good laugh now and then," quotes Alfred Berliner, the editor of *Die Naturwissenschaften,* as defining a scientific author as being "a cross between a mimosa and a porcupine," in fact, a *rara avis.*

The man who never writes papers may indeed be a paragon of knowledge, but he cannot escape some suspicion that he may not really have studied his lessons. When I asked Dr. Sam Harvey, then Professor of Surgery at Yale Medical School, if he would contribute a section on benign tumors of the breast to the *Textbook of Surgery,* which I was editing, he replied that he would be glad to as he "didn't know much about the subject." In other words, he would study and inform himself. I have published over a hundred papers, each of which has taught me something, and a few have been of importance; but they have all been the result of "mental sweat" and overtime work. Almost anyone can produce articles if he has the resolution to keep at it. Nothing annoys me more than the remark of many physicians, with a note of plaintive envy: "Oh, I wish I had the knack of writing!" Also to be deprecated were the words of a fine surgeon, who, although in one of Chicago's busiest hospitals, never wrote an article but said loftily: "I will never write anything unless I have something worthwhile to write about."

Every busy surgeon has unusual and instructive cases. The case report is the simplest form of medical paper. If accurately written and accompanied by a concise review of the pertinent literature, it is one of the cornerstones of medical knowledge. Alone or as part of a review of similar cases, it forms a real guide for practicing surgeons and for authors of textbooks. Nearly all surgical journals will publish worthwhile case reports.

In 1923 I attended a querulous 64-year-old business man who had had a rib resection for empyema performed under local anesthesia. Originating from this wound was a spreading carbuncular infection which caused him great pain. Despite many types of treatment by a succession of doctors, this virulent infection had spread widely. On the eighty-third day after his admission to the hospital, I was placed in charge of the surgical care. The carbuncular infection then extended from within 2 inches of the left of the umbilicus to within 3 or 4 inches of the midline of the spine. The upper level was the spine of the scapula and the lower level within 2 inches of the crest of the ilium. The problem was solved by ten separate operations under general anesthesia, each time a section of the necrotic infected skin being cut away. The patient left the hospital on the 139th day, completely recovered. The great medical artist Tom Jones made graphic illustrations of the condition and the method of cure, and my article was published in the *Surgical Clinics of North America* for June, 1924.

It was almost a "first." Unbeknown to me, Dr. Thomas A. Cullen, of Johns Hopkins, had an identical but much less severe case involving the abdominal wall. The publication of his case report occurred only about a month before mine, so he was rewarded with the honor of first describing this condition. He was good enough to write me on May 16, 1924: "It is particularly fortunate that I got mine out first because the case I reported in comparison with yours is like a side show to the main circus." Since then the condition has been observed and studied many times, particularly by Frank Meleney, of New York. Cullen is mentioned as the first to observe it, but usually my case is referred to also. Mester,[50] of Budapest, in 1940 said: "According to reports in the literature, Cullen was the first to observe the condition, after the removal of a suppurated appendix in 1924. The same year Christopher reported a similar process following rib resection for empyema thoracis." The condition was finally named "progressive postoperative gangrene of the skin" by Brewer and Meleney.

On another occasion I was a close second in describing a new lesion. In October, 1931, I[51] described a fracture of the anterior process of the calcaneus (heel bone). After my paper had been submitted for publication, I discovered that again I had lost out in priority, this time to an x-ray man,[52] who had published a paper in May, 1931.

In his most stimulating and valuable article on "The Physician in World Affairs," Trimble[53] aptly says: "Physicians' regard for human welfare transcends their nationalistic feeling." It is indeed moving to realize that men in all parts of the world are meeting the same problems of injury and disease which you are and are dipping eagerly into the great pool of medical knowledge, which gradually but inexorably transcends language barriers. The great medical libraries are the indispensable means of dispersing and sharing this information.

In 1936 I[54] published a paper entitled "Inflammatory Tumors of the Cecum Simulating Acute Appendicitis." In it I called attention to the fact that the surgeon who with good reason makes a diagnosis of appendicitis must be prepared occasionally to find a more serious lesion requiring extensive surgical correction. I reported a case of regional ileitis in a 31-year-old woman, requiring resection of the right colon; a case of carcinoma of the cecum in a 28-year-old man, requiring resection of the right colon; a case of diverticulitis of the cecum, requiring resection of the cecum and terminal ileum; and an abscess involving the cecum caused by Amoeba histolytica. Seventeen years later the medical librarian of the Evanston Hospital called my attention to the publication of a fine paper in the *British Journal of Surgery* entitled "Acute Phlegmonous Caecitis," by R. E. B. Tagart,[55] of Addenbrooke's Hospital, Cambridge, England. The opening paragraph of Tagart's article is as follows: "Frederick Christopher (1936) has drawn attention to four morbid conditions, which, though 'not often seen in the average surgical practice . . . stand out as a constant threat to all who enter the peritoneal cavity expecting to find pathology in the appendix only!' The diseases to which he referred were terminal regional ileitis, carcinoma of the cecum with abscess formation, acute caecal diverticulitis, and pericaecal amoebic abscess. The purpose of this paper is to draw attention to a fifth member of this sinister community." I wrote Tagart complimenting him on his contribution, which was beautifully illustrated in color, and he replied: "It was extremely kind of you to take the trouble to write, and a great encouragement to me."

In 1931 I received my first request from abroad for a reprint. It was from Dr. Giuseppi Pistocchi, in Bologna, Italy, who wanted a reprint of my paper, "Ileus Following Rib Fracture." This request was flattering and stimulating and at the same time was further support of the thesis that interest in medical problems is not limited to national boundary lines. Further requests for reprints or medical queries and comments came from Böhler, in Vienna; from Stettin, Germany; from Gutierrez, in Buenos Aires; from Leningrad; from the Royal Australasian College of Surgeons in Melbourne, Australia; from Ruthin Castle, North Wales; Amsterdam; Padova, Italy; Japan; Punjab, India; Leige, Belgium; Plovdiv, Bulgaria; Abadan, Iran; and Manila, Philippine Islands.

All in all, alone or with joint authorship, I published 128 papers. In addition to this there were also published reviews of some 75 books, of which 16 were foreign. Some of the medical papers were delivered before societies prior to publication.

In 1927 I began to prepare the manuscript for a book on minor surgery. Dr. Allen B. Kanavel kindly wrote a foreword to the first edition, which was published in 1929 by W. B. Saunders Company of Philadelphia. In the ensuing years I carried this *Minor Surgery* through six editions. The fifth edition was translated into Spanish (Espasa-Calpe, S.A., of Madrid, Spain). The seventh edition was published in 1955 under the joint editorship of Alton Ochsner, Professor of Surgery and Head of the Department of Surgery at Tulane University, New Orleans, and Michael E. DeBakey, Professor of Surgery and Chairman of the Department of Surgery at Baylor University, Houston, Texas.

Early in 1934 I assumed the editorship of *A Textbook of Surgery* (also published by W. B. Saunders Company of Philadelphia), which was comprised of contributions by various authorities in surgery. This textbook I carried through five editions, and by September, 1954, over 115,000 copies had been sold. The fourth edition was translated into Spanish in Mexico City (University Society of Mexico) and the fifth edition was translated into Italian by Dr. Maria Alesi Guarnieri under the supervision of Professor

Ettore Ruggieri, Director of the Surgical Clinic of the University of Naples, and published (1956) by Societa' Editrice "Universo," Rome, Italy. Dr. Loyal Davis, Professor of Surgery and Chairman of the Department of Surgery at Northwestern University, took over the editorship of the sixth edition, which was published in February, 1956.

Including the various editions of these two books and the Spanish and Italian translations, a total of over 200,000 copies have been printed.

The young surgeon must rigorously discipline himself to regular habits of medical reading. The best incentive to enlargement of his knowledge of medical literature is to "read up" on every condition encountered in practice. If he does not have ready access to a library, he must see that his textbooks are recent editions not obsolete. A loose-leaf "system" is of value to throw light upon a current professional problem. He may avail himself of the many "package libraries," which will be sent by mail by the American Medical Association and the various consultant and research services. He should always read the *Journal of the American Medical Association,* making a rapid survey of the abstracts therein, including those of other specialties as well as his own. He should subscribe to as many surgical journals as he can afford, including the *Annals of Surgery; Surgery, Gynecology and Obstetrics; Archives of Surgery; Surgery.* If he has access to an excellent hospital library with a generous file of bound periodicals, his problem will be much simplified, but he must regularly, preferably daily, be sure to visit the library. He must be thoroughly conversant with the value of rapid searching through the *Quarterly Cumulative Index Medicus,* and will be surprised how often he finds therein important information bearing on the solution of a difficult problem posed by some case which is troubling him. He is still more fortunate if the great libraries of a medical school and a privately endowed technical library such as Chicago's John Crerar Library are easily available. He will find his reading most interesting if he is trying exhaustively to cover all the literature concerned with a case or a group study which he intends to report. His mind will be far more enriched by a half hour in the library than the same time spent in jests, pleasantries and gossip in the doctors' lounge or coat room, even though the latter is entertaining and to a certain extent may invite referral of patients.

CHAPTER XI

Nonprofessional Activities

A N ACTIVE surgeon has little time for nonprofessional activities. To care for his patients conscientiously, to keep abreast of advances in his profession by reading and attending medical meetings, to earn his living, to care for and counsel his family, perhaps to teach in the medical school and perhaps to contribute to the medical literature are enough to claim all the time and energy of most men. However, it is to be hoped that there will be refreshing diversion. Richard C. Cabot was probably quite accurate when he named the four essentials to a man's happiness in his book, *What Men Live By,* as work, play, love and worship. We have devoted most of this book thus far to the subject of the surgeon's work. He must take time to enjoy the companionship and to be continuously on the lookout for ways of increasing the happiness of his wife and children and of others dependent upon him. The busy surgeon seldom can attend church regularly, but he must give the church his support.

I have come to believe that a surgeon's social relationships reflect his taste, and that no matter what types he most enjoys, nearly all of them are quite apart from any advancement in his profession. Indeed, they may be a deterrent to his progress. To me a few loyal, trusted friends with whom I can enjoy the benefits of informed conversation or perhaps a game of bridge or the like are far more enriching and diverting than a host of acquaintances. The competition necessary for success in newspaper-broadcast "society" is an exciting, rather ruthless and expensive pastime which has never appealed to me. This is fortunate, as I confess no talent in that direction. Large affairs are painful to me, and although one does occasionally see old friends for a few minutes whom one would otherwise rarely see, there is little chance for any real conversational exchange. The large country-club (more or less alcoholic) dances are enjoyed by many, but the intensity with which some persons try to project themselves back into the days of high-school flirtations presents pitfalls for the less wary or the more headstrong. The surgeon who figures largely in such parties may think he is cutting a dashing figure, but his conduct does not suggest to those whom he hopes to have as patients the picture of a surgeon with the granite-like imperturbability, clear head and cool judgment required in the operating room. His fortunes are further defeated if he falls into the error of casually entertaining a dancing partner with accounts of his surgical exploits, which may seem like subtle advertising to him, but as the identity of the patient will probably be recognized, it usually implants in the listener a warning that she does not ever want to be the subject for the entertainment of some other dancing partner. Patients should never be discussed at social functions, even when only doctors are present, for even though no names are mentioned, there is no assurance that identification will not be possible. A doctor's wife should never "know" whom her husband is treating or for what. A surgeon's wife preferably should not know the names of patients, for then she can more easily avoid embarrassing questions asked by her acquaintances.

While I enjoy a cocktail before dinner, I know most definitely that alcohol and surgery do not mix. A surgeon who is addicted to alcohol will be a failure. It is only hoped that such failure will occur early in his career and save many patients from his errors of judgment or of technique. I feel that the realization by doctors in general that alcohol and their profession are incompatible may explain the regrettable tendency of many of them when away from their work and at medical meetings to drink too much. When an average-sized man consumes one ounce of whiskey within an hour or less it is doubtful if his cerebral cortex is affected, and he has only a subjective feeling of warmth. His behavior is sociable and pleasant. But if the amount is two to three ounces, the alcohol in the blood becomes 0.05 per cent, and the cerebral cortex is affected. The inhibitions are weakened and judgment is blunted. He becomes boastful and impulsive, though while "high" he is still considered, more or less officially, sober.

The conventional cocktails served at dinner parties are becoming an increasingly difficult problem. The host and hostess desire to be hospitable to the nth degree, and the thirst of some of the guests may prolong the cocktail period for an hour or more. This is really a trying ordeal for the few who do not drink at all and soon tire of toying with tomato juice and listening to the laughter becoming louder. The cocktail is not only the enemy of good cooking, as the late Howard Vincent O'Brien once said, but after the high-calorie cocktails and "each-hostess-wants-to-have-the-best" appetizers, any interest for the real *pièce de résistance,* the actual dinner, is perhaps by nature's providence greatly reduced. The talk may be very lively; in fact, participated in simultaneously and even competitively. Under these circumstances it is no great strain to gain a reputation as a wit or to regard almost any anecdote as convulsively humorous. Many persons find this fun, but each to his own taste.

The surgeon must indulge in some sports and hobbies to refresh and divert himself. Those which get him out of doors and involve exercise are best but must vary with his age, physical capacity and individual tastes. Golf is a general favorite and fulfills most requirements with the additional advantage of good fellowship. It was never a success with me, however. I joined the Indian Hill Club when I was in the earliest and busiest stage of my career. Perhaps the frequent interruption by a caddy on a bicycle summoning me to take care of an emergency or perhaps my rather rotten game despite furious and intense efforts to improve it, was to blame, or perhaps I was more interested in other things. At any rate, in a few years I gave up golf and resigned from the club. I envy those who enjoy golf and are proficient in it. Earlier I played considerable tennis and got some exercise mowing the lawn, but I never really learned to garden.

The surgeon must get adequate rest, but the term "adequate" is open to dispute. Edison needed only a few hours of sleep at night (plus a possible nap or two during the daytime), and I suspect, but do not prescribe, that we need less sleep than we get. Serious surgical cases have caused me wakeful nights, but not infrequently valuable ideas have come to me during those times and I have implemented them by phone calls to the hospital. A certain amount of nonmedical reading is indeed restful. Biography has always interested me more than fiction, and the works of Winston Churchill have been read and re-read with relish. But after years of repeated experience I have found the best sleep-inducing book to be Creasy's *Fifteen Decisive Battles of the World,* which was re-issued in 1943, with nine additional battles described by Robert H. Murray, by the Military Service Publishing Company, of Harrisburg, Pennsylvania. After the physician's long hours of work and his considerable medical reading and, perhaps, medical writing, it is not surprising that his mind seeks light reading, such as detective stories, rather than more serious works for refreshment. Whitehead[56] observed: "In London I saw a good deal of physicians. After their day's work when they picked up their book or paper, they were too spent to think on what they read."

Although there is much truth in the maxim, "If you want to get something done, take it to a busy man," nonetheless it is only seldom that a successful surgeon will be able to find much time after his surgical work, teaching and writing to devote to civic duties. The nature of his profession, necessitating his being constantly on call, makes it impossible for him to be sure that he will have any given time free from interruptions. Local governments recognize this in exempting the physician from jury duty. In some instances it may be possible for a surgeon to hold a civic office, to serve on governing boards of various kinds, on Red Cross or other charitable committees, in Rotary or other organizations. In so doing he brings the broadening viewpoint of the physician to the group and also enlarges his own outlook. Sometimes he will be unjustly accused by colleagues of advertising, and sometimes they may be right.

In the current generation scarcely a doctor is to be found who has not at one time or another served in the armed forces. In performing this necessary and essential duty, he has usually done so at considerable cost to his professional development but never without some benefit to his character and social understanding. These periods of military service bring home to him the evil of war and should instill in him an awareness of the part he should play in decreasing it. In 1953, J. Ridgeway Trimble[53] gave a splendid address at the American Medical Association meeting entitled "Opportunities and Responsibilities of the Physician in World Affairs." He said, in part: "I would like to develop the following related thoughts: that only international understanding will prevent war; that physicians have a common language and enjoy the confidence of the people more than any other profession; that physicians know the true meaning of war better than anyone else; that politicians and statesmen and soldiers have thus far failed to prevent war; and that physicians have a great opportunity and obligation that they must seize and fulfill without further delay." While, certainly, physicians cannot alone prevent war, Trimble emphasizes that they have more influence than they suspect and it is incumbent upon them to exercise it to the maximum. Certainly the physician's function has a universal common regard and value despite a wide disparity of races and languages. Medicine is indeed a common denominator.

The surgeon should make appropriate contributions to charity from his earnings. I have little patience with the physician who proclaims that his good deeds are confined to taking care of charity patients. Actually, there is intense competition to secure a position as attending surgeon or physician on the staff of a large free hospital, for it is there that the surgeon inevitably acquires more proficiency and skill, which he call "sell" to his private patients. Or it is there that he can participate in research work or instruct students, which affords him enjoyment and increases his prestige. Charity work has its own professional reward, and it ill becomes a doctor to clothe it with an aura of nobility and self-sacrifice. What really counts is how much money he actually gives. The physician should contribute at least to the church, the Red Cross and the local Community Chest.

CHAPTER XII

Personal Injury Litigation

IT WAS a difficult problem for me to decide between the study of law and the study of medicine in my youth, and I have always been much interested in fundamental legal decisions and processes.

Surgeons must invariably care for patients who have been in accidents. The care of the injury in most cases is inextricably involved with the patient's real or alleged indignation at the other party concerned in the accident. "Get your money from him—it was his fault" is a common remark. It was told some time ago that a survey of x-ray examinations in accident cases at one of the Chicago hospitals showed that only 8 per cent had ever been paid for. The worst feature, however, is that many of the cases end up in personal-injury litigation. The waiting period before the trial may be several years, during which the patient (and his attorney) must not allow himself to forget his sufferings. In fact, the agony caused by the accident occasionally seems to increase, and not infrequently the patient's recovery to well-being is actually retarded. While, of course, many of the cases are of a serious nature and it is the doctor's duty to describe the injury as objectively and accurately as possible, many injuries are trivial, being magnified by the patient for the purpose of obtaining a large settlement at the trial.

In one case in which the injuries had occurred three years before I was put on the stand to testify and were of such a minor nature that I could not remember them, the patient's attorney pointed his finger at me and shouted fiercely: "Did she have a bump on her head?" Because of its frequent dishonest use, the expression "I do not remember" seemed to me something I should avoid at all costs, although in this case it certainly was the truth. Fearing I might do her a wrong if she had had a bump and I did not remember it, or if she had not had one and I said she did, I would hurt the defendant, I pondered the answer. Finally, I came forth with what seemed to me a most sagacious reply: "Well, she might have had." I was startled at the general laughter, even from the judge, which my remark evoked.

A rude awakening for the young doctor is caused by a subpoena. Up to the moment that this harsh, unfeeling hand of the law has been laid upon him, he has felt himself to be a free agent, each day involved with the heavy responsibilities and unscheduled calls of seriously ill people. But the attorney also thinks he himself is busy, and, as the law is on his side, he can compel the surgeon to come to court. If you do not do it graciously, the lawyer can punish your lack of cooperation by keeping you for long periods in the court- room—may even secure a "bench warrant," which keeps you there on call. Several years elapsed before I abandoned my naive idea that, if I could avoid a subpoena, I could escape going to court. Never was there a more fallacious idea.

Perhaps I had paid too much attention to the yarn told about Dr. Coleman Buford at the old Alexian Brothers Hospital in Chi- cago. One day while operating in the single-doored operating room, Dr. Buford was told that a process server was waiting outside to serve a subpoena on him when he came out. Buford completed his operation, lay down upon a cart, had himself thoroughly draped with sheets and wheeled out past the process server, much to the delight of the doctors and nurses.

My final recognition of the futility of trying to avoid a subpoena came about after my learning, on one occasion, that I was likely to be subpoenaed in a minor accident case. While sitting at dinner one night I received an unusual phone call from the local druggist, who said he was sending over a patient who had inquired of him the directions to my house. This ruse seemed to me so superficial that I refused to open the door to this "patient." The next morning while I was in the operating-room suite at the hospital, I was told that there was a patient downstairs anxious to see me. I asked to have the patient come to the telephone and inquired about his symptoms. When he said he felt bad "all over," it seemed to be almost certain that he had a subpoena in his hand, so I referred him to another doctor. When he said, "But, Doctor, I have confidence only in you," my choler completely overcame my judgment and I made some regrettable statements, concluding with the altogether treasonable and childish remark: "And if you ever do succeed in getting me down to testify, you'll be sorry you ever did." These dire happenings were reported to the judge with, I have no doubt, flourishes, exaggerations and emphasis. The next thing I knew, a slightly embarrassed, polite but none the less determined armed sheriff came from Chicago to Evanston, found me in the hospital and placed me under arrest. He drove me to Chicago and brought me to the courtroom, where the trial was in session. The judge looked thunderclouds at me, and for the first time I began to reflect that perhaps this was going to be serious. Contempt of court was punishable, especially when a judge looked as angry as this one did. I was put on the stand and qualified, and the attorneys for the patient began to shout loudly at me: "And you said it would be too bad for us if we did get you down to court!" After my testimony, which was not important at all, the judge turned his mind to my misconduct. He regarded me long, silently and with extreme disfavor. I hoped I was not going to jail. Finally he said, "Doctor, you know we expected better things of you. I will fine you the cost of the sheriff's trip to arrest you—four dollars." I concealed my relief as I paid my fine. Once more I could breathe the beautiful free air of Chicago!

The men who usually represent the plaintiffs—the personal-injury lawyers—do not seem to be chosen from the ornaments of the legal profession. A pencilled note that I prize was written by a patient on whose behalf I was to testify and delivered to me while I was sitting in the courtroom one day. It read: "Dear Doctor: I regret your having to come into a sordid matter of this kind. A man of your profession should not have to spend time away from the sources where he does so much good. . . ."

In 1927 I[57] reported two unusual cases of multiple fractures. One of these patients was a man of forty-nine who was brought to the Evanston Hospital after a train accident in which he sustained twenty-eight separate fractures and lost a leg. While still in a critical condition, he was visited by a personal-injury attorney and interviewed. The attorney assured the apathetic patient that he would fight for his financial interests, but this necessitated setting down all the facts connected with his case. The lawyer would have to "talk to the landlady of the house where the patient roomed," and as she would not know who he was, would the patient please sign this little "note of introduction." The patient signed what he later found to be a contract engaging a certain law firm to represent him. I became incensed at this misrepresentation and appealed to an attorney friend of mine. He brought the matter before the Chicago Bar Association's committee, but no action could be taken as the culprits were too skillful in protecting themselves. When the final settlement was made by the railroad, the signed "note of introduction" secured half of the money for the disreputable law firm, although another firm, one of high repute, had done all the work.

About this time I took care of a woman who was injured while riding in a taxicab. She sustained a relatively minor injury of the neck—a fracture of two of the cervical vertebrae without any paralysis. The treatment, however, was not minor, as I had to place her in a plaster cast to hold her head, neck and shoulders rigidly. After the cast was removed, I had her wear a firm leather shoulder cape, from which was supported by many adjustable turnbuckles a leather collar supporting the head. It took the weight of the head off the fractured bones of the neck and was rather comfortable to wear. Its appearance, however, was indeed dramatic, for it resembled some strange torture engine of the Middle Ages. After she had worn it for a number of weeks, its use was discontinued. I discharged the patient from the hospital when her neck was virtually painless and she had about 98 per cent of normal motion. A few months later I learned that the patient's husband, the proprietor of a poolroom on the west side of Chicago, had returned to the hospital and had obtained the formidable-looking neck brace from the supply room, where it had been stored. Somewhat concerned that she might have had a relapse, I telephoned the husband, who said: "Oh, don't worry, Doc. She's O.K. But her trial begins Monday, and she has to have the brace to wear to court!" When I appeared at the courtroom, having of course been subpoenaed, I found the jury assembled in the jury box, reading newspapers and glancing occasionally at the tragic figure of my patient, wearing the leather brace and grimly turning her head, neck and shoulders as though they were in one piece. The attorneys were "in chambers" trying to settle the case out of court. The attorney for the patient realized that he had a strong card to play just by exhibiting the patient in her brace. Although the patient's hospital and doctor bills had not exceeded $500, her attorney was putting on strong pressure. He would come out from time to time to report his progress in the struggle, and I was astonished to hear that he "had them up to $10,000." Later it was $12,000, and the patient said to her lawyer, "Aw, let's take it. I'm tired of being what I ain't." I never have understood why the defending attorneys did not let the case go to trial, put me on the stand and ask, "Does she have to wear that brace?" My answer in the negative would have collapsed her case. However, my patient's attorney announced that we were all going to lunch "on him." Late in the afternoon the case was settled for $18,000, and her attorney did not seem displeased with his share, $9,000, for his day's work.

W. L. White,[58] in an excellent article entitled "The Personal-Injury Racket," tells of a newspaper report of an early-morning collision of two street cars. By noontime thirty-four persons had presented claims for injuries sustained in that accident, not knowing that the newspaper account had omitted mention of the fact that one of the cars was empty and returning to the car barns and that the other was a repair car, carrying no passengers.

CHAPTER XIII

Surgical Fees

THE subject of surgical fees is a difficult one. The patient does not wish to have an operation and often does not have insurance or savings to cover the unexpected and unwanted costs. The surgeon, on the other hand, has had costly education and training and is usually over forty before his surgical practice provides much of an income. He has his family to provide for, is expendable in a sense and must attempt to provide for his later years, as a surgeon seldom continues remunerative activity as long as an internist does. Usually, the subject of fees is not discussed in medical school, most medical teachers seeming to think it a somewhat unmentionable and hush-hush subject, not to be discussed with eager young students, who presumably devote their thoughts exclusively to the study of medicine and guard themselves from the sordid idea that they must eventually support themselves and their families by the practice of medicine. For my part, I have often discussed fees with interns and residents and have never failed to find them keenly interested and usually most woefully uninformed. Advice and information on this subject may save them from alienating many patients and may provide a policy and plan which will give them more time for the purely intellectual and professional aspects of medicine.

The matter of fees is involved and changes with any variations in the economic well-being of the country and with the more general utilization of health insurance plans, such as the Blue Cross, and even such extremes as the complete socialization found

in Great Britain. Michael Davis[10] says: "We can be fairly certain that fee-for-service payment by the consumer of medical services will continue to diminish. It constituted some 85 per cent of all expenditures for medical care in 1929 and had fallen to 60 per cent in 1951."

Long experience has made me feel that the following observations can be of value to the young practitioner. Contrary to the notion which is sometimes expressed that a man's competence is judged in the patient's eyes by the fee he charges, in general a physician does himself far more harm by overcharging than by undercharging. There are very few individuals, indeed, to whom medical expense is not a real and often serious matter. I do not deny that there are occasional patients of great weath to whom a large fee is a matter of little moment, but that same fee would constitute a real hardship to most persons. Let no young doctor harbor the illusion that he can treat only wealthy patients; there simply are not enough of them. Furthermore, a wealthy man immediately recognizes an overcharge and resents it. In the long run, the offending doctor is harmed far more than he is benefited by the one exorbitant fee.

A doctor who is obsessed and preoccupied with professional earnings can never succeed and is harmful to the profession. However, a businesslike awareness of charges is expected by the patient and when the amount is tempered by mercy and kindness, he is most appreciative. Undue delay in sending bills is usually annoying to patients. When, despite the fact that a charge has been made with thoughtfulness and kindness, the patient asks for a reduction, this may be proper. If the patient prefaces such a request by genuine appreciation of the medical services and by sincere explanation of his own financial difficulty, the physician should usually reduce the bill. But when the patient starts his request for a reduction by stormily declaring that the services were not worth the price and that he was grossly overcharged, the doctor is, humanly, much less likely to grant a reduction. It is therefore of first importance that daily charges be made with careful, conscientious thought and that the total bill should be reconsidered before being rendered.

On one occasion I was consulted by a woman who asked me the cost of removing a wen from her scalp. I replied: "Oh, five or ten dollars," at which she announced that she would take the five

dollar operation! However, she still seemed to worry that I might charge her ten, so during the operation under local anesthesia her conversation was directed principally in the hope that I would charge only five dollars, giving the following amazing reason: "You know, my husband hasn't worked for a year and he is getting so nervous that we are going to have to take a Mediterranean trip and therefore must be careful of our expenses."

On another occasion a wealthy woman, accompanied by her elderly housemaid, came to the office to discuss the arrangements for an operation which the maid needed to have. The "conversation" was for the most part a monologue by the employer, with frequent emphasis that the maid had been with them for many years, that she "was like one of the family," and that they wanted her cared for like one of their children. Finally silence prevailed, so I knew that the subject of the fee was about to be broached. Sure enough, the hitherto silent maid timidly asked, "What will you charge me, Doctor?" The employer, to say the least, was prudent.

Many years ago, an employee of one of my friends was advised to have a leg amputated at the hospital on the West Side of Chicago where he was a patient. Nothing would do but that I should see this patient and have a consultation with his surgeon. The consultation was a mere formality, as the man's leg was gangrenous and had to come off. The patient's wife asked: "What do you charge to take off a leg?" I replied that it was $150. By that time it was well after midnight, but this obviously poor family went into a prolonged, worried huddle. The result was that they called up Dr. Edward Ryerson, one of Chicago's leading orthopedic surgeons. It was a cold night, and Dr. Ryerson could not have been in the best of humor to be wakened by the telephone and abruptly asked "How much do you charge to take off a leg?" He gruffly replied, "Four hundred dollars," and the family chose him! Certainly, since his price was so much higher, he must be a much better surgeon! Parenthetically I may mention that on three occasions I was paid several hundred dollars more than I had charged—a most heartwarming experience.

Dr. William S. Thayer, of Johns Hopkins, used to tell his graduating classes: "Have one regular charge for each of your different services and reduce it when the patient's circumstances warrant it." This is merely another way of saying that the patient's ability to pay should be related to the fee. While this principle seems proper and

ethical to me, it is bitterly attacked in some quarters. Howard Whitman[59] has said: "Soaking the rich for medical care is a device of the fee-gouger today. It springs not from social justice but from greed. If one of the biological blackmailers ever tells you, 'But this enables me to do other work free of charge—for charity,' just ask him, 'In what other business or profession does a man insist that his charity be paid back at the next rich man's expense?'" I do not feel that these harsh remarks are justified. A wealthy man—and after all there are not very many these days—may find it much less of a hardship to pay $50 than would a man on a small salary to pay $10 for the same service. Moreover, many men of higher income are prone to think that if the charge were $10 the service would be a fifth as skillful or valuable as it would be if the charge were $50. I know of one wealthy man who reproached an internist for referring him to a young surgeon who said he would charge $15 for removing a wen. "I don't want any $15 man!" he told the internist. The latter replied: "You must have misunderstood the surgeon. He must have said $50. Go and see him again." This the patient did, but before he could get there, the internist telephoned the surgeon and told him sternly: "You said $50!"

In Chicago, some sixty years ago, Dr. N. S. Davis annoyed his fellow practitioners by charging uniformly only $1 for an office call. Dr. Herrick[60] in his most interesting autobiography relates two episodes regarding Dr. Davis:

"Dr. I. N. Danforth told me how a patient from Dakota came storming into Dyche's drugstore at the corner of State and Randolph streets and asked if there was not some other doctor than N. S. Davis to whom he could go; he had not come to Chicago to see a one-dollar doctor. Mr. Dyche advised him to 'go upstairs in the same building and consult Dr. Danforth.' While the man was climbing the two or three flights of stairs, Dyche whistled through the speaking tube that communicated with Dr. Danforth's office and told him the circumstances. Dr. Danforth reported to me: 'I gave that man a good honest, thorough examination and the best advice I was capable of. I charged him twenty-five dollars. He was satisfied and—so was I.' . . . There was a well authenticated story that once Dr. William H. Byford was asked by a lady how he could charge her three dollars for consulting him in his office, while Dr. Davis charged her only one dollar. Dr. Byford quietly replied, 'Madam, I am not responsible for Dr. Davis' fees, but I assume he knows the value of his own services better than anyone else.'"

The courts have considered the matter of adjusting the physi-

cian's fee to the patient's ability to pay. The Supreme Court of Iowa (Robinson vs. Campbell, 47 Iowa 627)[61] stated the belief that the value of a service depends on the skill required in its performance, and sometimes on the results accomplished, but not on the riches or the poverty of the person for whom the service is performed, and this court said: "There is no more reason why this charge should be enhanced on account of the ability of the dependents to pay than that the merchant should charge them more for a yard of cloth, or the druggist for filling a prescription, or a laborer for a day's work." However, the Supreme Court of Texas (Caulk vs. Anderson [Texas], 37 S.W. [2d] 1008) took the opposite view, saying:

> "Since a cardinal object of a physician's employment is to prolong the life and restore the health of a human being, any evidence bearing on the pecuniary value of such life and health cannot be logically ignored in search for the truth as to reasonable compensation for the services rendered under the employment. The principle which must govern in this case is the principle that underlies the settled rule in negligence cases, that in ascertaining the pecuniary loss resulting from death or permanent bodily injuries, the jury may consider, not only the age, occupation, habits, and health of the deceased or injured person, but also the amount and value of his property and his earning capacity. Had the patient (Brackenridge) suffered permanent injury or lost his life as the proximate result of the negligence of his physician in performing his professional duties, no one could question that he, or a dependent relative, might have proved the patient's wealth and business capacity, under the established law of Texas, in an action to recover the damages for which his physician would then have been liable. Such testimony would be admissible because it would help to determine the pecuniary value of the patient's health and life. For the same reason, testimony of a patient's wealth is admissible as a circumstance to determine the value of services resulting in the restoration of his health and his capacity to perform his customary duties, as well as in the prolongation of his life."

An authority on medical jurisprudence says: "In most states, though, the patient's financial status is *not* a legally admissible factor in fee determination. In only a handful of states (e.g., New York, California, Louisiana, Missouri, Pennsylvania and Washington) have courts held that a physician may properly consider the patient's income when setting the fee."[62]

No one questions that it is entirely proper for a lawyer to fix his fee in relation to the amount of money involved in a case. It

124

may require exactly the same, or nearly the same amount of legal knowledge and of work to set up the articles of incorporation for a small corporation with $100,000 capital as it does for a huge corporation with $100,000,000 capital, but no one questions the propriety of the attorney's fee being much higher in the case of the larger corporation. The doctrine of the consideration of the client's wealth or poverty in the determination of the attorney's fee is in accord with the opinion of Associate Justice Grier[61] of the Supreme Court of the United States. (Lombard v. Bayard) who said:

> "Every gentleman of the bar well knows that there cannot be any one rule of charges in the nature of a horizontal tariff for all cases. Often, where the parties are poor and the matter in contest is small, counsel receive but very inadequate compensation for their exertion of body and mind; and for myself I know that for some of the most severe labor of my professional life I have been least well paid. In other cases, where the parties are wealthy, and the sum in controversy large, they will receive a tenfold greater compensation for perhaps a tithe of the same labor. In some cases the whole sum in dispute would be poor compensation. In others, five per cent of it will be very liberal. Hence, in all cases, professional compensation is gaged not so much by the amount of labor, as by the amount in controversy, the ability of the party, and the result of the effort. And this is perfectly just."

According to Maurer,[63] the average gross annual income of physicians is $24,000 and the average net income is $14,300. The estimated present cost of medical training is $22,000. The general practitioner's net income averages about $8,000 and specialists average about $15,000. Of the specialists, the average net income is highest in orthopedic surgery ($18,000) and in roentgenology and radiology ($17,500) and lowest in internal medicine ($12,500) and pediatrics ($12,000). The average number of hours per week worked by doctors in all fields is fifty-seven and ranges from forty-four for the dermatologist to sixty-two for the pediatrician.

According to Whitman,[59] some fifteen thousand doctors display in their waiting rooms plaques obtained from the American Medical Association which read: "To All My Patients—I invite you to discuss frankly with me any questions regarding my services or my fees. The best medical service is based on a friendly, mutual understanding between doctor and patient." I was always pleased when a patient asked me the cost of an operation. I am still amazed at the hesitation and embarrassment exhibited by some in bringing the matter up, and I fear many inexplicably lack the courage to do it. A glib, confident demand may betray the "shopper," who goes to several surgeons trying to get the lowest price. This type, however, is infrequent, and most patients are sincerely interested in trying to see how an unwanted expense can be fitted into their budget.

The patient may open the discussion of charges by the flat question: "Doctor, what will your fee be?" or, "How much is all this going to cost me?" My reply to this question is according to one of the following methods:

The first method is to state my customary charge for the operation, if it is a standard one. For example, $200 for a hernia or $350 for a gallbladder operation. Several years ago when the prices of food and clothing were half what they are now, those figures were $150 and $300, respectively. Somehow or other, professional fees lag behind the rise in living costs. When a flat sum is mentioned, it is always qualified by some such phrase as "barring unexpected complications which might require additional professional care."

The second method of reply is used when you do not know whether the patient is on a small salary and is making a formidable financial sacrifice to have the operation and is too proud to refer to it, or whether he is a relatively prosperous man. In the former case, I would be inclined to quote a fee somewhat lower than customary. I then say: "The expenses involved in this operation come under three headings: The hospital, the special nurses and my own fee. The hospital cost will vary with the hospital and the type of accommodation. A bed in a 4-bed ward costs $17 per day, and in a 2-bed ward costs $19.75 per day, either of which is completely covered by a "comprehensive" Blue Cross policy. The private rooms vary in cost from a few at $22 per day to $35, with an average of $27. Additional charges are made for the operating room, anesthesia (often a separate bill from the doctor administering it), laboratory fees and unusual medicines. I expect you to be in the hospital for six to eight days."

At this point the patient may interrupt and say, "Doctor, my financial circumstances are such that I must take the very cheapest accommodations." Or he will say, "I must have a private room." At this time it is wise to tell the patient that while you will ask for the type of reservation he has requested, he must not be surprised to find that when it is time for admittance to the hospital a series of unpredictable emergency admissions will oblige the hospital to give him something less desirable. As to special nurses, it may be that the operation is of such a type that I have been able to say, "Special nurses are not mandatory. You would have more attention with special nurses, but the 'floor nursing' will be adequate. The cost of the three eight-hour shifts for full coverage of special nurses is about $50 per day. Special nurses are difficult to obtain; many more could be employed if they could be found, so that you must not be surprised not to find one ready on the morning of the operation, even though a 'booking' was made one or two months ahead of time." As in the matter of the type of hospital accommodations, the patient may here interrupt to say, "I simply cannot afford special nurses!" or "I must by all means have full coverage, day and night."

With information as to the patient's preferences and his financial ability to take care of them, the doctor is now in a much better position to state the fee he will charge. He will be able to sense that a charge perhaps less than his regular one will be indicated. Or he will find that the cost is not of too much importance to the patient and that the size of the fee may have some relationship to the patient's estimate of the surgeon's skill and experience.

Those patients who most anxiously inquire about the doctor's charges can usually be most depended upon to pay their bills. Whenever a patient says: "Spare no expense, Doctor!" it may mean that he is not interested in the slightest since he has no intention of paying. When the doctor feels that his charge will be a real hardship for a hard-working person with a small salary, he may give a lower figure immediately. But the doctor is rightly annoyed when, because he has been impressed by a patient's stringent need of a ward bed and has fixed his fee accordingly, he finds that the patient finally takes a private room. Such a patient may feel that he has shrewdly reduced the doctor's charges and can put the money saved into fancier accommodations at the hospital. In other words, the doctor is really paying for the more expensive room! Sometimes the patient will sheepishly remark: "Oh, Aunt Kate gave me a present of the money for a private room." Although I have never done so, I can understand why some doctors at the outset say that their fee will be a certain amount if the patient is in a ward bed, that it will be a larger amount if he is in a private room and a still larger amount if he has special nurses.

The third method of reply to the patient's query about charges for the operation is one I have been using more in recent years, especially if the operation is one which will require protracted after-care with many dressings. An example of this type is obstructive resection for carcinoma of the left colon, a type of operation which is, to some extent, being supplanted by primary resection. Here there is a temporary colostomy, much detailed advice and wound care are involved and the whole postoperative period lasts for possibly two months. To the patient, "an operation is an operation," and his limited knowledge of the costs and the amount of work involved may be based upon casual conversations with acquaintances. If you say $500 before the work is done, the patient may feel that the charge is high (because his neighbor had an "operation" for $250). On the other hand, if he receives his bill after he has seen how much work is involved and what the surgeon's services have meant to his comfort and recovery, he will seldom protest at the charge. These considerations bear on the development of my third method of reply. The answer is "I do not know at present what the charge will be, as I cannot predict with accuracy the amount of work I will have to do. When I have completed my work and you are discharged as a patient, I will send you a bill which I believe to be fair and proper. *If, however, this bill is not suited to your financial circumstances, I will ask you to name the charge and that will be it.*" Note that it is pointed out that the patient may name the fee if the doctor's charge is not in accord with the patient's financial circumstances, but *not* if he considers the doctor's work to be worth less. I have used this method many times and have never regretted it. On the few occasions when a patient has requested a reduction of my charge, there has been no complaint of my work but an explanation which has invariably been satisfactory to me as to why the fee would work genuine hardship on the patient. In requesting a smaller figure, no patient has ever taken an unfair advantage of my permission to have him name the fee.

I am inclined to think that young surgeons particularly are likely to make errors in charges. As they gain in experience they will be much less likely to make errors, which can result in loss either of friends or of justly earned income.

Written on one man's bill for $200 was the note: "My wife and I are deeply grateful for your skill and devotion and the fine results of your work. I am ashamed to send you a check, as the charge is absurdly low."

Another man was sent a statement for $75, and on it I wrote: "This is just a suggestion. I really don't know what you would think suitable. Send whatever you want to, and I will call it square." He sent $75 and replied: "This is the first time a doctor has given me the option of deciding the amount of the bill. It is a pleasing privilege. Based on the time devoted to my case, I had estimated your charge would be $50—which I thought fair. But your way of leaving it up to me is so considerate and liberal as to discourage argument."

From a grateful woman: "I just must tell you how happy your bill made me today—that sounds odd—being happy over a doctor's bill, but we knew we couldn't afford your services and yet just couldn't be content with anyone else. I was more unhappy over putting my husband under the burden of debt again than over the operation. But your kindness has not only left us hope of that first vacation in eight years, but your consideration for our circumstances has brought a warm cheer and we want to thank you for it."

A surgeon is supposed, generally, to *do* something visible or mechanical for his money. Mere counsel, such as an attorney gives, often seems to the layman to be noncompensable. One time I was surprised to get a note enclosing a check for $50 for thoughtful advice to a man, since I had not sent him a bill. The note read: "In appreciation of the counsel and service given us for which you have not sent a statement."

Fee splitting is a secret deal between a surgeon and a family physician in which the former rebates to the latter a part of the fee collected from the patient for an operation. The evil lies in the tendency for the family physician to find the surgeon who will give him the largest rebate, rather than to find the surgeon who will do the best surgical work. Moreover, there is a temptation to form dishonest teams of family physicians and surgeons to promote unnecessary operations. In the present state of perfection of surgical technique, such operations can be done with little risk to the patient, who is none the wiser. The first line of defense against this pernicious practice is the quality of the standards at the hospital where the operation is done. All surgical work should be an open book; all tissues removed should be reviewed by an honest, fearless pathologist and/or committee; and the hospital should have at least 60 to 70 per cent of the hospital deaths covered by necropsies.

The public has been warned against the evils of fee splitting and unnecessary surgery. The many devious procedures of fee splitting and how the public may be on guard against them were fully described by Steven M. Spencer in the *Saturday Evening Post* for January 16, 1954, in an article which carried the endorsement of Dr. Paul R. Hawley, Director of the American College of Surgeons. The October 30, 1953, issue of *Colliers* carried a story with the lurid title: "Why Some Doctors Should Be in Jail." The article entitled "Unjustified Surgery," by Greer Williams in *Harper's Magazine* for February, 1954, notes that public opinion was so aroused that "The North Dakota legislature passed a law requiring all surgeons to notify the clerk of the county court and get the approval of two other doctors before every operation, and afterward to deposit with the clerk as a matter of record whatever was removed from the patient." The governor vetoed the measure because, as Williams says, he was "unwilling to see county courthouses become museums of either normal or pathological tissue."

Williams quite properly says: "Hospitals which live up to the requirements of the Joint Commission on Accreditation of Hospitals (JCAH) are the public's best assurance that surgery will be dependable, although rascals pop up even in accredited hospitals. The essence of their requirements as they apply to surgical care of the patient may be summarized in four R's—responsibility, rules, records, and review." Responsibility refers to the duties of the governing board to insure the best staff and the highest standards. Rules are those laid down by the staff, with the sanction of the board, for its own conduct. Such rules should empower the proper committee to determine what surgical privileges, if any, a doctor may have. Myers,[64] an administrative assistant of the American College of Surgeons, says: "The determination of surgical staff privileges is probably the most difficult and important decision which confronts the medical staff of any hospital." Myers suggests minimum standards for what he terms "full surgical privileges" and "limited surgical privileges." He proposes a system of "medical audit" of the hospital practice of every physician, both medical and surgical. The third R deals with records. In all hospitals it is necessary to have a records committee to insure the keeping of full and up-to-date records. Such a committee should be backed up by hospital authorities so strongly that doctors who are delinquent in the matter of records will be denied hospital privileges. The fourth R deals with review. All surgical departments should have weekly or at least biweekly reviews at which the operations and surgical deaths are discussed.

The Columbus Surgical Society[65] has carried the war on fee splitting a step farther. In its by-laws it states:

> "There shall be an annual audit of the professional records and accounts of each member of the Society, including income tax returns. The accountant or auditor shall be designated and instructed by the Council. . . . The examiner's report shall be strictly limited to the data showing the presence or absence of fee splitting as defined above. Each member of the Society shall supply the examiner with whatever waiver or permit he may need to conduct the above examination and to permit him to report his findings to the Society. . . . Failure to permit the audit shall be construed an irregularity and sufficient reason for investigation . . . and disciplinary action."

The society retains the accounting firm of Ernst & Ernst and in the first two years turned up three men who were using two sets of books, one for the society and one for income tax purposes. The Columbus plan has been taken up and followed in one form or another in Bloomington, Illinois; Indianapolis; Detroit; Lincoln, Nebraska; Brooklyn, New York, and Iowa. On November 12, 1954, the Chicago Daily News reported that "members of the medical staff of Michael Reese Hospital announced yesterday they have requested that institution's board of directors to approve their voluntary agreement to disclose their income tax returns to prove they do not split fees. A spokesman said the action was taken as a preventive and not a curative measure, because fee splitting has never existed in the hospital." The staff president said that the new system "will reassure the public that doctors' ethics are above criticism."

On August 23, 1956, the Supreme Court of Ontario, Canada, dismissed the attempt of three London, Ontario, doctors to have the Victoria Hospital's anti-fee-splitting by-law declared invalid. The three doctors objected principally to the by-law which enabled the hospital to have a staff doctor's books audited and gave the trustees power to deny doctors the privileges of the hospital. Mr. Justice LeBel said that the patient is entitled to assume that the doctor who recommends an operation has no pecuniary interest in it. He said that, while the practice is not forbidden by the Criminal Code of Canada, nonetheless in his opinion it is illegal.

While actual fee splitting is still difficult to uncover, at least it is openly attacked by the best members of the profession and is rarely present in the best hospitals. The surgeon, however, will have to be on guard constantly against the more subtle maneuvers through which an internist may strive to get more financially out of an operation. The glaring fault of fee splitting is that the patient receives only one bill and does not know how the money is divided between the surgeon and the internist. Sometimes only the surgeon's name will appear on the bill, but he will rebate a percentage to the internist who referred him the case; or, what is slightly less pernicious, the names of both men will appear on the bill but the proportion that each is to receive is not indicated. Another form of pressure on the part of the internist is to send a separate bill in a pure and open manner but to try to dictate privately to the surgeon what his bill should be. The internist may say: "This patient has $500 to spend on this operation. The hospital bill will be about $150. You charge $250 and I will charge $100 for the diagnosis and some visits afterwards." The honest surgeon, of course, must make his fee entirely in relation to his evaluation of his services and to some extent, the patient's income, but he will have to be resolute and independent in the face of this thinly veiled threat on the part of the internist, even though he knows that failure to fall in with the internist's plans may mean that the latter's next patient will be referred to another surgeon.

My own feelings on this matter will best be shown by the following actual correspondence with a prominent internist, whose name will of course be withheld:

"January 31, 1951. Dear Dr. Christopher: The report of the operation (which you sent me) on Miss ——— brought to mind a matter of considering of finances. I judge that she is wholly responsible for her own bills, and that being the case I would suggest that you and I get together and decide upon a figure that will be satisfactory for both of us. You realize of course that Dr. ———, my assistant, and I will have put in about the same amount of time as you did in managing the case and therefore a bill will have to be rendered by you and us that will be in a sense equitable. Yours very truly,"

I replied:

"Dear Dr. ———: Thank you for your letter of January 31st in regard to Miss ———'s finances. I, too, thought she should be given some consideration. Accordingly, I have decided to send her a bill for $400, which is $100 less than I might otherwise charge. Of course, you and Dr. —— will have to decide yourselves what bill you consider proper."

I do not think that thereafter I was referred a single case by this man unless a patient had definitely requested my services. Fortunately in the better hospitals these influences are minor, but they are mentioned here for the young surgeon's guidance. In most instances the surgeon's skill, kindness and fairness in the matter of charges are the factors governing an internist's referral. The patient will often ask the internist: "What will the surgeon charge me?" I much prefer to have the internist tell the patient that I will be fair but that the patient must discuss this matter with me directly, preferably before an operation.

CHAPTER XIV

Imponderable Rewards

of Surgery

To the young man considering the study of medicine, to the young practitioner often weighted down with onerous and unpleasant duties and to those unconnected with the practice of medicine itself, a consideration of the imponderable or spiritual rewards and satisfaction of the physician may be enlightening.

The first type of reward is the entirely impersonal and purely intellectual satisfaction of finding and evaluating the evidence of disease, of making a correct diagnosis, of choosing the correct or optimum treatment and of seeing this treatment produce the anticipated results. Such satisfactions are not dissimilar from those associated with evolving a new and more efficient piece of machinery, with the construction of a legal instrument designed to serve multiple long-term purposes, with the solution of a mathematical problem or with completion of some literary work. While it is true that diagnosis and therapy, to be successful, require the physician's intense interest, there are some in whom this interest is so great that it tends to make them increasingly impersonal. While physicians with the purely intellectual approach may give the highest type of service to their patients, they are prone to be impatient or even annoyed with human foibles, emotions and ignorance. I have seen doctors with the highest intellectual attainments who are unable to secure their patients' confidence and co-operation.

A second type of reward is that of manual accomplishment, of seeing the results of the use of the hands which only long practice and increasing skill have made possible. Such satisfactions are those of the surgeon who surveys a completed resection of the right colon before closing the abdomen, or who views the x-ray of a highly successful reduction of a difficult and complicated fracture or who inspects the improvement in a patient after plastic surgery has corrected an unsightly defect. Such satisfactions are no doubt akin to those experienced by an artist upon completion of an oil painting, by an architect when he sees the finished house his mind has fashioned on paper, or by an engineer who gazes on the finished span of a bridge which he has designed. Satisfaction in manual skills must be sought by the surgeon particularly, but if they are his only or predominant concern, he can never achieve distinction. He tends to become an "operator," albeit a skilled one. His technical achievement becomes his chief objective, rather than a means of gaining his main objective—the patient's improvement.

The third type of reward comes in research. Here is the intellectual fascination of probing and hunting for the unknown. Search of many blind alleys, infinite patience, and fortitude in disappointments are involved in the adventure. Techniques may have to be learned and then discarded when found to be impracticable or useless. Many delicate tests must be endlessly repeated. The researcher faces daily the strong possibility that his work may lead to nothing. But, hovering over him are the shadowy examples of Roentgen, of Curie, of Fleming. Some workers seek fame, some yearn to lighten the burden of mankind's suffering, but all of them have the sustaining enjoyment and excitement of the hunt. Those who find their greatest happiness in such efforts should, for the most part, be in great institutions of research, and society should make it possible for the relatively few who are gifted in this way to give their full time to research and to be free of financial worry. The latter requirement should be met easily, as most of these devoted individuals have relatively simple material wants. The research worker seems to be constituted entirely differently from the practicing physician, and the latter is dependent upon the results obtained by the researcher.

Of course many instances could be cited in which a busy practitioner, with a flash of intuition or inspired appreciation, has discovered or devised some improvement in medical diagnosis or therapy. Moreover, there is the almost limitless field of clinical research to which men in active practice can always contribute. Painstaking study and impartial analysis of methods of treatment help greatly in the evaluation of those methods. In a sense, *every* practitioner should be a contributor, provided his records are carefully made and periodically reviewed.

The research worker is often much involved with animal research. Without vivisection, medical progress would be stopped. To me it seems entirely proper that the lives of mice, guinea pigs, rabbits and dogs should be humanely sacrificed in order to save the lives of human beings. Incidentally, animals themselves are often benefited by the advances in knowledge made possible by vivisection.

The fourth type of reward, and to me the most satisfying and important of all, is the human satisfaction—to see a patient relieved of pain, to see health and hope return. Inextricably bound up with this reward is the satisfaction derived from a patient's expression of gratitude, which is usually verbal. Rewarding also are the eloquent thanks expressed by a patient's relatives; the grateful look from frightened parents when their child's injury has been repaired or an operation successfully accomplished. Probably no words are spoken more sincerely than those of a grateful patient to his doctor. Words of gratitude are spoken daily, and they warm the doctor's heart, spurring him to carry on although fatigued. Every doctor knows this, but he can seldom recall just what was said, the inflection of the voice or its depth of emotion.

The *written word,* however, can be read and re-read. Just what does a patient say when he is deeply grateful? How does he put it on paper? Words differ with the depth of the emotion involved and with the individual's educational background, but the common denominator is *sincerity*. A patient is not competent to appraise the skill required for an operation which, in a given case, may not have been too demanding, but his words of gratitude depict the skill as it appeared to him, its recipient. Moreover, a surgeon is usually praised more often than an internist, because the surgeon's services are often rendered at an especially critical moment and frequently are of a serious and dramatic nature. The general practitioner who cares for numerous, often minor ailments for many years in the same family has loyal regard and respect, but is, perhaps, less likely to be the recipient of letters of praise.

It has seemed to me that reading some of these expressions would have a heartening influence on students and physicians and on patients and relatives, themselves. I do not know that it has ever been done before, and this is indeed understandable, as doctors who receive letters of gratitude are modest about them. These letters are private, and the doctor abhors putting himself in the position of "blowing his own horn," of advertising or of painting a glowing picture of himself. Because of these factors, a great quantity of precious human material is lost; precious because of its inspirational nature to those contemplating the study of medicine and those plodding in the traces of daily practice; and precious because it helps others realize what these feelings are and how they are expressed. The distinguished philosopher, Alfred North White-head,[56] has said: "I think you get a truer picture of a period from intimate letters written spontaneously and without a thought of publication than you do from its fiction and often better than from its historians." And Harvey Cushing[66] quotes Southey's dictum that "a man's character can more surely be judged by those letters which his friends addressed to him than by those he himself penned, for they are apt to reveal with unconscious faithfulness the regard held for him by those who knew him best." Moreover, it is not inappropriate in these times, when so much sensational material is being published dealing with unworthy members of the medical profession, to read some of the words of appreciation which patients have addressed to a doctor.

Accordingly I have decided to quote anonymously parts of some of the letters I have received from grateful patients. I have saved over a thousand of these letters and have pasted them in scrap-books. They bring back vivid memories of battles with disease and injury, and of the courage and fortitude shown by the patients. I have now retired from all professional activities, so I can not be accused of advertising, and it is certainly not my intention to be boastful. The reader is asked to keep in mind that the following letters are merely given as examples of what most doctors receive but keep to themselves.

A letter from a prominent Chicago attorney, whose wife I had operated upon for a severe tendon-sheath infection resulting from a wound made with a can opener, included the following words:

"Mrs. —— and I both feel that you saved her life and that we shall both be grateful to you as long as we live. Words cannot express our appreciation of your skill, devotion, patience and resourcefulness."

A recent patient wrote:

"I appreciate so much the modesty of your bill, which is a real help to me at this time. I only wish I were a wealthy woman that I might more materially evidence my thankfulness for your skill—tho' I feel, too, that nothing could ever quite fully express it all."

The father of a four-year-old boy upon whom I did *not* operate (despite the recommendation of an eminent pediatrician) and who subsequently developed typhoid fever, an incident which I have described previously, wrote:

"There is really no way that my wife and I can really tell you of our appreciation for what you did for us. We have spoken of it many, many times together and with deep gratitude for your judgment and courage. Of course, such things are common in your daily existence and it must be the biggest satisfaction of your profession, but a single instance like that leaves an indelible impression on us to whom it means the most. With this you have the gratitude and appreciation of Mrs. —— and myself. We are very thankful that your prompt action and accurate diagnosis saved the day."

One night I went to the house of the "high-powered," irritated and suspicious president of a large Chicago corporation, who tried (unsuccessfully) to block the steps I took to operate upon his son, who was seriously ill with severe acute appendicitis. I prize the letter the father later wrote:

"Looking back over the recent experience with our boy, I am impressed with the fact that your handling of the situation was no ordinary service. I can now see more clearly that, besides the illness, you had to deal with an obstreperous boy and a doubting and excited father. To know that your diagnosis was correct—that your patient has gained six much-needed pounds since the operation, and that the father has returned to normalcy should give you much satisfaction. We will never forget the decisiveness, firmness and skill which you displayed and will always be thankful to you."

From a doctor whose daughter I operated upon:

"Although it is impossible to express one's full appreciation in writing, I feel that I must tell you of our feelings toward you because of the splendid service rendered our daughter. Many times in the past we have faced crises of various kinds with our children but never before with such confidence. A doctor's family is often the worst neglected medically because no one cares to assume full responsibility. Your quick decision and action lifted the task from the shoulders of a doctor-father whose judgment regarding his own child is necessarily biased."

In childish penmanship, from a doctor's daughter, whose cut tendons I sutured:

"I am sending you this program to let you know that I can play the piano. Paderewski may play it better, Levine may play it louder, and Harpo Marx may play it funnier, but not with more satisfaction. You will remember that you spent a hard afternoon sewing together all of the cut tendons on the top of my left arm following an automobile accident."

The following humorous letter is from an attorney friend on whose wife I had done a cholecystectomy:

"My wife says you are a wonder and that the operation was a complete success. I am not so sure that I agree. I had counted on getting a glimpse of my bride once or twice during a leisurely convalescence, but as far as I can see, there was no such period. She didn't miss a single social engagement and was . . . again running all over the country, apparently from the very moment you withdrew the knife! Anyway, here is my check, but if, when I finally do catch up with my bride, I find there is no scar, and there was no operation, then I want my money back!"

Also when death occurs, the expressions of appreciation from the family are usually verbal. It has been my custom to write a letter of sympathy to the bereaved family. The doctor, better than almost anyone else, can write such a letter, for during a terminal illness he is closer to relatives and knows more of the details and facts than anyone else. Three general themes seem to help the family and lighten their sorrow. First, they are always appreciative of words of admiration for the deceased, particularly a child, and for the gallant fight he put up. Second, they need reassurance that no stone was left unturned to save the patient's life. This may or may not include specific or general recapitulation of the steps in the treatment and the reasons for making them. It may also delicately summarize the autopsy report. And, third, it is almost always possible to thank the family for their cooperation, patience and understanding, and to praise their loyalty and devotion to the loved one who died.

The following quotations have been selected from letters received from relatives of deceased patients:

From a widow:

"Your letter has been one of the greatest consolations in my sad hours. You were more than kind to write, and it is with the deepest appreciation from myself and the family that I write these few lines which so feebly express what I feel. . . . When all earthly sources fail, we still have the everlasting arms to lean upon and I am sure my dear husband is by our God and Savior's side helping me to carry on."

From a young widow in Oklahoma, whose husband died of peritonitis from a ruptured appendix, which at that time was a far more perilous condition than now:

"Your good letter of a week ago received the first of this week and I know not how to express my deep gratitude to you. . . . With so many loving relatives, new and old good friends and strength given by God I have been able to keep going. . . . I really wish you might have known my husband when well. He surely did admire you and it was our whole family faith in you that kept us so well. We knew not what to do at times but you were always so kind when we knew well you had many other patients and their families to comfort too."

From the mother of a fine young doctor who died of a malignant disease:

"My husband and I have never forgotten your kindly consideration for us when we were with _____. There is a very deep satisfaction in knowing that all was done for him that the best minds knew. He felt that comfort himself and often said so. During all his months in the Evanston Hospital you were instrumental in giving him courage. He told us how secure he felt in your hands. His optimistic attitude made everything easier for himself and all of us, did it not? He is a wonderful son and we are rich in memory. Please accept the sincere gratitude we feel in our hearts for all you did for him."

From a man whose wife I cared for in a fatal illness:

"I have been wanting to write you for some time, but have not been in the mood to do it until now. I do want to express to you my sincere thanks and appreciation for your many kindnesses shown to my wife and myself during her long illness. She had great confidence in you and I know her many visits to the hospital to see you were made more pleasant by your kind and personal attention to her, and the exchange of friendly repartee between you had much to do to buoy up her spirits. Your sympathetic interest in your patients is an outstanding characteristic seldom found in men of your profession and is indeed something in which you well may take great pride."

Epilogue

THE achievement of a satisfying surgical career is not easy. Unremitting mental and physical drive and patient fortitude are vital in overcoming discouragements, but these qualities, of course, are the same as those which are necessary for success in practically every field of endeavor.

All doctors are rewarded by deep spiritual satisfactions. In the case of the surgeon these are particularly clear and impressive. All who contemplate the study of medicine, or those students of medicine who are considering surgery as a specialty, should be given every encouragement and hope. There is much to be done; there is room for many.

References

1. Major, Ralph H.: A History of Medicine. Springfield, Ill., Charles C Thomas, 1954.
2. Finney, J. M. T.: A Surgeon's Life. New York, G. P. Putnam's Sons, 1940.
3. Osler, William: Aequanimitas, and Other Addresses. Philadelphia, P. Blakiston's Son & Co., 1904.
4. Fabricant, Noah D.: Why We Became Doctors. New York, Grune & Stratton, 1954.
5. Rosen, George, and Caspari-Rosen, Beate: 400 Years of a Doctor's Life. New York, Henry Schuman, 1947.
6. Mayo, William H.: Proc. Staff Meeting, Mayo Clinic, March 30, 1932.
7. Severinghaus, A. E.; Cadbury, W. E., Jr., and Carman, H. A summary of their report is given in Time, Nov. 2, 1953.
8. American Medical Association, Council on Medical Education and Hospitals: 56th Annual Report on Medical Education in the United States and Canada. Journal of the American Medical Association, *160*:1637, Aug. 25, 1956.
9. Gibbon, John H., Jr.: Presidential Address before the American Surgical Association, Philadelphia, Pa., April 27, 1955. Transactions of the American Surgical Association, *73*:1, 1955.
10. Davis, Michael M.: Medical Care for Tomorrow. New York, Harper & Bros., 1955.
11. Clark, Donald M.: New England Journal of Medicine, *251*:137, 1954.
12. Means, James H.: New England Journal of Medicine, *250*:766, 1954.
13. Journal of the American Medical Association, 1956.
14. American Surgical Association: Report of the Committee on Graduate Surgical Education. Annals of Surgery, *138*:937, 1953.
15. Naffziger, Howard C.: Annals of Surgery, *140*:261, 1954.
16. Spencer, James H.: Bulletin of the American College of Surgeons, *39*: 119, 1954.

17. The present secretary of the American Board of Surgery is Dr. John B. Flick, 225 South Fifteenth Street, Philadelphia. See: Journal of the American Medical Association, *159:*479, 1955.
18. Cope, Oliver: New England Journal of Medicine, *250:*1, 1954.
19. McKittrick, Leland S.: New England Journal of Medicine, *251:*61, 1954.
20. Beecher, Henry K.: Journal of the American Medical Association, *151:* 44, 1953.
21. Elkin, Daniel C.: Bulletin of the American College of Surgeons, *42:*5, 1957.
22. Means, James H.: Doctors, People and Government. Boston, Little, Brown & Co., 1953.
23. Jordan, Edwin P.: New England Journal of Medicine, *250:*558, 1954. The Physician, His Business and His Practice, Boston, Little, Brown & Co., 1954.
24. Burrows, Harold: Pitfalls of Surgery. New York, William Wood & Co., 1925.
25. Garland, Joseph: The Physician and His Practice. Boston, Little, Brown & Co., 1954.
26. Hall, George E.: Legal Aspects of a Medical Partnership. Journal of the American Medical Association, *156:*1312, 1954.
27. Jordan, Edwin P.: The Business Side of Group Practice. Journal of the American Medical Association, *155:*1371, 1954.
28. Hamilton, Walton H.: The Place of the Physician in Modern Society. Quoted by Curtis, Charles P., and Greenslet, Ferris: The Practical Cogitator, Boston, Houghton, Mifflin Co., 1945.
29. Homans, John: Obituary. New England Journal of Medicine, *251:*240, 1954.
30. Wartman, William B.: Quarterly Bulletin of Northwestern University Medical School, *29:*69, 1955.
31. Slee, Vergil N.: Bulletin of the American College of Surgeons, *39:*397, 1954.
32. Myers, Robert S., and Slee, Vergil, N.: Bulletin of the American College of Surgeons, *41:*109, 1956.
33. Lembcke, Paul A.: Journal of the American Medical Association, *162:* 646, 1956.
34. Myers, Robert S.: Bulletin of the American College of Surgeons, Nov.-Dec., 1953. See also: Myers, R. S., and Stephenson, G. W.: Evaluation Form for Tissue Committees; Suggested Method for Tabulating Decision as to Justification for Surgery, Journal of the American Medical Association, *156:*1377, 1954. Daseler, E. H.: Bulletin of the American College of Surgeons, *40:*22, 1955.
35. Myers, Robert S.: Bulletin of the American College of Surgeons, *41:* 173, 1956.
36. Regan, Louis J.: Medicine and the Law. New England Journal of Medicine, *250:*463, 1954.
37. Cole, Warren H.: Bulletin of the American College of Surgeons, *41:*67, 1956.
38. Bulletin of the American College of Surgeons, *39:*152, 1954.

39. Myers, Robert S.: Bulletin of the American College of Surgeons, *41:* 207, 1956.
40. Gilchrist, Richard K., in discussion of a paper by West, John P.: Cardiac Arrest During Anesthesia and Surgery. Annals of Surgery, *140:*623, 1954.
41. Koontz, Amos R.: Journal of the American Medical Association, *156:* 1629, 1954.
42. Potts, Willis J., as reported in the Chicago Tribune on March 16, 1955.
43. Cole, Warren H., and Sadove, Max: Journal of the American Medical Association, *162:*437, 1956.
44. Beecher, H. K., and Todd, D. P.: Annals of Surgery, *140:*2, 1954.
45. Bulletin of the American College of Surgeons, *41:*126, 1956.
46. Crossen, H. S., and Crossen, D. F.: Foreign Bodies Left in the Abdomen. St. Louis, C. V. Mosby Co., 1940.
47. Morrison, R.: British Medical Journal, Feb. 9, 1924, p. 255.
48. Bulletin of the American College of Surgeons, *41:*441, 1956.
49. Einstein, Albert: The World As I See It. New York, Philosophical Library, 1949.
50. Mester, A.: American Journal of Surgery, *47:*660, 1940.
51. Christopher, F.: Journal of Bone and Joint Surgery, *13:*877, 1931.
52. Dachtler, H. W.: American Journal of Roentgenology, *25:*629, 1931.
53. Trimble, I. R.: Journal of the American Medical Association, *153:*1143, 1953.
54. Christopher, F.: Inflammatory Tumors of the Cecum Simulating Acute Appendicitis. Surgical Clinics of North America, *16:*215, 1936.
55. Tagart, R. E. B.: Acute Phlegmonous Caecitis. British Journal of Surgery, *40:*437, 1953.
56. Dialogues of Alfred North Whitehead, As Recorded by Lucien Price. Boston, Little, Brown & Co., 1954.
57. Christopher, F.: Multiple Fractures. American Journal of Surgery, *2:* 422, 1927.
58. White, W. L.: The Personal-Injury Racket. Reader's Digest, Jan., 1955. See also Regan, L. J.: Malpractice, an Occupational Hazard. Journal of the American Medical Association, *156:*1317, 1954.
59. Whitman, Howard: Woman's Home Companion, July, 1953.
60. Herrick, James B.: Memories of Eighty Years. University of Chicago Press, 1949.
61. Journal of the American Medical Association, Feb. 20, 1932.
62. Swetlow, George I.: Medical Economics, 1954.
63. Maurer, H.: The M.D.'s Are Off Their Pedestal. Fortune, Feb., 1954.
64. Myers, Robert S.: Bulletin of the American College of Surgeons, *39:*69, 1954.
65. Williams, Greer: The Columbus Plan Begins to Roll. Bulletin of the American College of Surgeons, *39:*153, 1954.
66. Cushing, Harvey: The Life of Sir William Osler. Oxford, Clarendon Press, 1925, Vol. 1, p. 128.

Index